# This is Reiki

# This is Reiki

The book that has inspired thousands of Reiki practitioners

Arístides Molina

First Spanish Edition: June, 2006

Second Spanish Edition: June, 2013

Third Spanish Edition: June, 2019

Copyright © 2006 - 2019 Arístides Molina

https://estoesreiki.com

ISBN13: 978 1 0711 0100 1

# DEDICATED

To Migo,
To my earthly family,
To my students and colleagues,
To the family "I am".

# CONTENT

# ACKNOWLEDGMENTS

To Wilda Soto Aguirre, for believing in me and take my hand, undertaking a challenging path filled with amazement, setbacks and conquests, but always new and beautiful.

To Marinela Ramírez, for her trust, her friendship and her support to this project and others we have shared. Thank you!

To Nekane de Leniz To Mimi Urrunaga and to Beatriz Lozano, my partners in Canal de Luz, Peru. Thank you for your companionship, your friendship and devotion.

To my dear and beloved students, with whom we have shared laughter and tears… this book would not have existed without them.

To Silvia Yadira Ladera Castro, my spiritual partner, a companion of quests and encounters, for her unconditional support to almost any of my "follies."

To all Masters of Reiki. To my lineage and especially to my Usui Tibetan Reiki Master, Jaime Oli-ver P.

To my conscious teachers as Paramahansa Yogananda and Osho. They know why.

To all masters from other realms as Kryon, Serapis, The Group, Kwan Yin, Tobias and Saint Mi-chael the Archangel. Thank you for your infinite wisdom and compassion.

To the Source, to my Higher Self and to my Guides, for allowing me to live this human experience and for illuminating my path.

To my whole I AM Family,
Thank you.

# PREFACE TO THE FIRST EDITION

Many years ago since my early beginnings with my conscious learning journey of Tarot and Vi-bration Therapies, I heard about Reiki Energy. At that time I thought this was a very complicated therapy for me, that it was going to take too much of my already limited time. At that moment I thought this was more consonant with Massotherapists, with Traditional Chinese Medicine Schol-ars, as well as, "cabin" healers; while I preferred a more mental, psycho-spiritual work toward guidance. I used to read about the subject more ou: of curiosity than interest of an apprentice, tak-ing some general information for reference only. That it has been called "general culture".

Twenty years later I met Aristides Molina, and initiate a rich chain of synchronicities that took us to share different roles and joint experiences. During the last year we have been a teacher of the other, fellow workers and associates in publishing projects. His teachings are more of sharing life knowledge, going beyond his authority in holistic and complementary therapies, which place him in a role of a reliable and qualified teacher. It is always a delightful and instructive time listening to his comments, conclusions and contributions. And there is no doubt about how inspiring is to share his concerns, projects and paradoxes.

This work you are about to read is the result of years of investigation, learning and life. It is not just the work of a very dear friend but as well the one of a teacher from whom learning is always present. This is Reiki is the result of the systematization done by Aristides Molina during a long time, as a means for transmitting to his students part of his experiences during his journey, as well as new contributions, images and other contents.

It is written with the love a master can only pose on his teachings and with the devotion a guide places just to facilitate those following the path. Here it is the importance of the mission he has accepted to comply with this publication. This is not just a book written to be published and com-mercialized but a book with the intention and desire of communicate, sharing a decanted and lived knowledge. Now after being published and available to the big public, it becomes a lighthouse, a mentor and a invaluable resource for learning. In this book you will not only find the Reiki Princi-ples, as well as its objectives and procedures, expressed with simplicity and depth, but also the experiences lived by an acute and diligent therapist, the synthesis of years of road traveled and lived experience. Those who have ventured into this vast knowledge by other means, will find in this work many answers to their questioning, a more inspiring application of Reiki, and also a guide so clear and orientating that becomes a text about Reiki of a mandatory consultation. For those who do not know about this inspiring healing path, This is Reiki, will place at their fingertips a guide to start a path of ascension.

Reiki is a way of feeling and sharing, giving and receiving love, and healing. But above all, it is a way to praise and experience the love from the infinite Light Source. In that sense, this is more than a book about Reiki, it is Reiki itself.

Finally, when mentioning Reiki one has to include its creator, Mikao Usui, then I have to make a comment regarding the headstone placed by his students few years after his death. It reads that he was a good working man, humble and of a strong build and always with a smile in his face. He was a talented man, with a taste for reading and a deep knowledge about History, Medicine, as well as various spiritual and esoteric disciplines… What a parallelism! How to best describe the author of this work?

Namaste.

Lic. Marinela Ramírez
Founder of Superior School of Tarot

# AUTHOR'S NOTE

Before anything, I would like to write few words about Reiki.

To study Reiki is something very simple and it takes few hours to know the practice and to re-ceive the energy tuning. Living Reiki is a spiritual experience for life. In my case in particular, it has changed my life in such a way that I don't remember a single aspect that has not been touched by this subtle and wonderful energy. Reiki works silently and constantly making changes in us which in many cases are miracles. More than a healing technique, Reiki is really a gift, a divine dispensation for our species, for the Planet and for the whole Universe.

It is a genuine pleasure for me to share this Reiki experience with you.

Dunas

*Reiki con intención*

*no tiene límites,*

*Reiki sin intención*

*es una oportunidad desperdiciada.*

# WHY ANOTHER BOOK ON REIKI?

There are many books about Reiki available in Spanish but I have not heard that there is one written by a Venezuelan. While that would be a good reason to publish it, it is not the only one

Writing this book, ruled by Tibetan Usui Reiki, is a way to honor what the practice and experience of Reiki have given me over the years. Reiki has been a great partner in my life and a great help when facing different process of self-knowledge, self-assessment and inner peace, which otherwise would have been impossible to overcome.

Of course I will not repeat what I have found in other manuals received from my teacher. Neither will I repeat what has been said in other books of the same subject. While some of the content is unavoidable and will be similar in all the books of Reiki, much of the above here is the result of my experience and intuition, faculty that has developed noticeably with my experience with Reiki. This book is, essentially a result of the maturity of my relationship with Reiki. What has allowed me to expand my understanding, open up to other content, finding new and interesting relationships between different concepts, and so enhancing my perception of what this technique means.

I do some emphasis on the energy aspects of Reiki, to make explicit the energy unit of all that exists, showing how Reiki is inserted and related to the whole. Spiritual things are not divorced from the material and therefore may be analyzed with a kind of reason-intuition we might call spiritual logic. This is a very handy resource at a time when all our benchmarks of faith have failed we are unbelievers.

The spiritual logic is proposed in this book enables you approach the Reiki not only as a belief but also from the highest planes of conscious understanding. This approach to understanding the technique can make the difference between using Reiki or not do, in those difficult moments when everything fails on faith. It is a way of telling the Reiki practitioner does not need to believe in Reiki since there is a foundation of this technique works, beyond belief and devotion.

# ABOUT ENERGY

Everything that exists is energy, so it is impossible to have a precise definition, because our minds cannot encompass the whole, even in imagination. In the absence of a definition, man studies energy through its manifestations. Thus were characterized through Science, different types of energy. As an example we can mention gravitational energy; electromagnetic energy and nuclear energy.

Quantum physics has reached a point where they recognize that the matter is not different from the energy, but energy is in a state that is perceived as matter. For more than 30 years physicists create matter "from scratch", from energy, using linear accelerators. Ironically, it is one of the largest machines built by man, several kilometers, designed only to study the microworld.

Beyond the energy types recognized by science, there are more subtle ones that have been recognized and utilized by different cultures through the ages. Chinese talked about Qi (Ki for the Japanese), defining various types of energy as the Ancestral Qi, the essence, and the acquired among many. The subtle energy that animates life is called Prana by Hindu people. In Western, a similar energy is known as Orgon, Odic Foce and Astral Light.

The Human Aura is formed by the energy of subtle bodies, invisible to the common human eye, like: the etheric, the emotional or astral and mental. There are modern sophisticated devices attesting these energies, like Dermatron, capable of measuring the etheric body and, Kirlian camera that is capable of showing the human aura. There are other less sophisticated tools like the pendulum and dowsing rods that allow interacting with the human auric field. At least part of the energy of these subtle bodies is electromagnetic, with a vibration difficult to detect with conventional devices.

Recently, Dr. David R. Hawkins, PhD, psychiatrist and researcher was able to measure conscious levels using kinesiology technique. One of his most recent results is a scale that facilitates the study, understanding and evaluation of conscious levels in persons, objects or events. This discovery verifies the old paradigm that everything is energy, including subtle aspects of consciousness. Later we will explain in more detail some relevant aspects of this discovery.

## Properties of Energy

Both in Science and Spirituality, Physics and Metaphysics we have used many models to describe the nature of energy, While none of these models are incomplete, each serves to intellectual or intuitive approach to those aspects of the energy we want to highlight.

One of the most used models to represent energy, from the point of view of physics, is the wave model. It has been applied very successfully to study sound behavioral aspects; electromagnetic energy (brain, radio, TV waves; microwaves, infrared waves, visible light, ultraviolet, X-rays, and so on), as well as micro-particles. It has also been very useful in my teaching Reiki to convey some crucial properties of energy that can be a bit difficult to communicate.

The chart presents a summary of some of the fundamental properties of energy explained by means of waves.

Let's study these properties, one at a time:

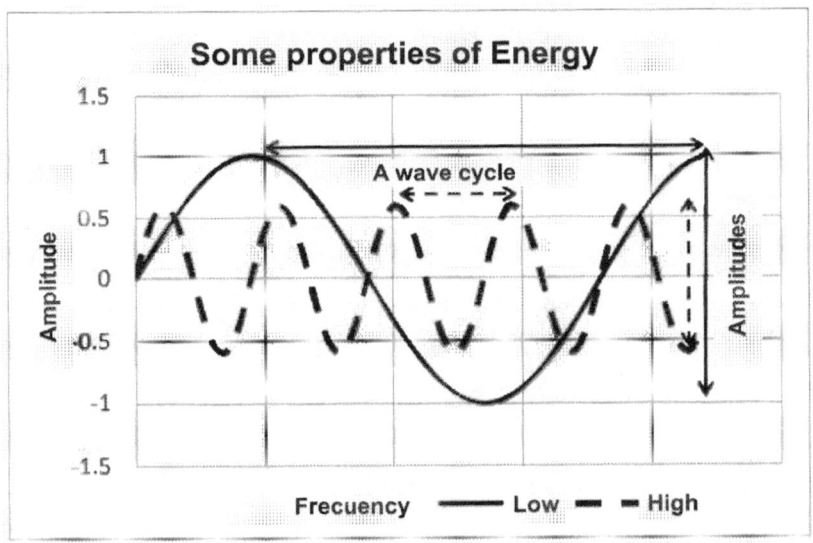

## Oscillatory Aspect

The two waves have a portion of the graph above and one below zero. The top portion can be identified as positive: Yang, masculine, day, summer; while the lower part is related to the negative: Yin, feminine, repose, night, winter. Both portions are the same energy. It is a unit expressed in this plane oscillating between opposite polarities. One cannot exist without the other, just there is no Yang without Yin, day without night, rest without activity.

It is vital to understand this characteristic of the energy because it saves us the sterile belief that that there may be something called positive energy away from its negative counterpart or vice versa. The same is extended to the concept of good and evil that is wielded both when looking at things from the angle of ethics. There is no good separated from bad. The two aspects: Yin and Yang exist only as aspects of the underlying unit of which they are an integral part. There are not two things, there is only one thing that can be seen as dual under certain circumstances and with certain level of consciousness.

## *Frequency*

It is the number of times a wave repeats itself in a given time. Usually, it is expressed in Hertz (Hz), in honor of the German Physicist Heinrich Hertz. One Hz is one cycle per second. Wave with the solid line in the graph has a frequency higher than the dashed line, ie having a higher vibration.

Frequency measures the power of energy; the higher the frequency, the greater the energy. In the electromagnetic spectrum, radio frequencies (10 Hz to $10^9$ Hz) are practically harmless. However, somewhat higher frequencies of ultraviolet (greater than $10^{15}$ Hz) damage the skin and X-Rays (greater than $10^{17}$ Hz) can cause infertility and severe diseases.

Sounds are also frequencies, as with musical notes. For each note of each octave corresponds to a fundamental frequency that, in the case of central A in piano it is 440 Hz. The audible frequency range is between 20 Hz and 20 KHz approximately, where lower frequencies are bass sound and higher frequencies to the treble.

In the field of consciousness, Dr. Hawkins has characterized the different levels under physic-mathematical terms, with a scale of frequencies measured in Hertz. Thus, shame is a vibration frequency of $10^{20}$ Hz, while anger vibrates at $10^{150}$ Hz and at $10^{540}$ Hz joy. Anger is of lower frequency than joy. Thence, anger is an emotion that lowers our level of consciousness while joy increases it. What is sometimes known as negative energy is nothing but low frequency or vibration energy. And the so called positive energy is just high frequency energy. All vibrations, low or high, have a positive and a negative aspect to manifest in duality. Later in this book, is discussed in greater detail this discovery and its special relationship with Reiki.

## Amplitude

The Amplitude is indicative of the number of "items" with the same frequency. If we talk about light, the amplitude of a beam of red light tells us the amount of red light photons are emitted. The amplitude is perceived as intensity of said light.

The sounds we listen in the radio are a set of frequencies simultaneously perceived. The amplitude of these sounds is not simply the volume of the radio. If we lower the volume to zero, we get no sound so none of the sound frequencies is expressed. And as we increase the volume there is greater amplitude for each frequency.

Likewise, at a behavioral level, if I am a little angry, my anger amplitude is less than if I am really angry. Anger is a frequency that with certain amplitude is perceptible – I know I am angry.

However, the magnitude of the amplitude can make a difference in my behavior. A greater amplitude in anger means that anger has blinded me and I am prey to anger. If anger amplitude is zero, it means that there is absolutely no expression of such energy.

## Non-destructive co-existence

Each and every frequency can expressed itself at each space-time point. That is, each space-time point is a container capable of bearing all frequencies at once. This means that, in theory, all frequencies are everywhere but many of them have zero amplitude therefore not expressed and not perceived.

Radio waves are a good example. In the same radio equipment, using exactly the same antenna, different frequencies can be heard, even different frequencies bands such as AM and FM. Sounds and music are also a good example of this property of energy. Each instrument has a different timbre, which is nothing else than the simultaneous combination of frequencies and amplitudes that occur when executing each note. The music and choral arrangements are examples of how man has learned to use to their delight this non-destructive coexistence of different frequencies.

In people, this principle is very well observed in the coexistence of different frequencies ranges or bands corresponding to the physical, emotional and mental in the same human body. Even within the vibratory levels of the physical body, each organ handles a particular frequency spectrum. A non-destructive coexistence is also evidenced in the mixture of feelings and emotions we continually experience when combining different conscious levels.

## *Harmony*

Harmony is a property of the energy that talks about the natural concert or affinity of the frequencies and the intrinsic relationship between them. When various frequencies are expressed together in harmony, the result is almost always perceived as something nice.

In the case of music, the paradigm of energetic harmony is clearly expressed through the relationships between the different sounds of the scale. A chord is an example of harmony that combines various sounds or frequencies. The harmonic combinations of chords are based on the natural relationships between frequencies or harmonics generated by using a musical sound.

A natural C chord is built with the most relevant harmonics that occur when issuing note C. Harmonics are integer multiples of the fundamental frequency of C. In this case they would be: fundamental frequency or tonic f - C; a higher octave tonic 2f - C; dominant 3f - G that originates a fifth Interval; a two higher octaves tonic 4f - C; 5f - E originating a third Interval.

Successive harmonics, although there are expressed at lesser extent, that is, they have much less amplitude than the aforementioned. On this occasion, a natural C chord is composed by C, G and E notes, which are the most relevant harmonics of note C.

At levels of consciousness usually happens something similar. Anger and fear are often closely related, like joy and peace. It is clear that the harmonics knowledge of conscious levels is not so systematized as that of music, nevertheless, there is evidence of harmonic relationships between them.

## *Resonance*

Resonance is the fundamental mechanism of energy's interaction at all levels. Simply put, can be explained as the synergistic effect that occurs when two energies of identical or similar frequencies meet each other.

This synergistic effect results largely in the amplitudes of the two frequencies are combined and complimentary, creating a high current energy (amplitude) for said frequency. Usually, the resonance, left on its own, tends to increase indefinitely until one of the bearers of such systems often collapses. That was the case with the Tacoma Bridge, in the United States that collapsed on November 7, 1940, as a consequence of 68 Km/hour moderate winds. Structurally, this bridge had frequencies very similar to the energy generated by the wind. The bridge, began to oscillate slightly at first but by maintaining the wind-down frequency, the amplitude of its oscillation increased in such a way that destroyed the bridge.

But Resonance is not destruction by itself but only the synergistic effect between different systems with identical or similar frequencies.

Resonance is an interacting way between people as we also are energy, as are our thoughts and emotions. If you express anger to a person, it is likely the person expresses anger to you, unless it is someone consciously able to make their own choices. If you express joy, joy you will receive. If you just simulate joy and this is not your fundamental vibration, others will feel it in some way and will act accordingly, consciously or unconsciously.

Knowledge of this property shows us that we are responsible of circumstances in our life. Our perceptions, at every level are made possible by the existence of resonance. We see, touch, smell and feel by resonance.

Emotionally, we only resonate with those frequencies built-on us. So our anger, for example, it is not due to anything external but to have that kind of vibration within ourselves and allow that to be amplified, either by direct contact with said frequency or as harmonic of other emotional vibration akin to anger.

If things are left on their own, we will always be easy prey of emotional tides. But if we become aware of what is happening, without passion, we can consciously change the course of events and set off our lives on the path we choose.

## Analogy

Analogy is another crucial aspect of the energy and refers to a special kind of harmony and resonance. As we have seen, there are other type of energies like electromagnetic, gravitational, emotional, sound, mechanic, thermal and many others. An energy of a given type can stimulate, regulate and serve as reference to another type of energy thus promoting its organization.

Take the case of colors and sound. There is a fairly clear analogy between these two types of energy, which related the red with the note C; the orange with the note D and so on. These two energies are in turn related to the human biology in different ways. One of them is through chakras.

Thereby we can use energy systems such as color or sound to regulate and stimulate other type of system, analogous to those, which is the chakra system. However, if we look at the similarities of the Five Elements of Chinese Cosmology, we find that we can use colors and sounds in a different way, to stimulate vital energy, organs and emotions.

Another case of analogy is the energy of aromas. This is a type of biochemical energy, that is, electromagnetic, capable to stimulate other type of energy such as emotional and mental. The analogy is also one of the fundamental mechanisms of the mind so that is akin to the power of thought. .

## Analog Harmonic Resonance

Although already discussed above, it is important to summarize the issue about energy interactions by presenting the basic mechanism of all energy interactions.

The interaction between all things in the Universe is based on a principle called Analog Harmonic Resonance. While this is not the only principle that defines and encompasses such interactions, it is valid to explain how it occurs. It is a systemic global vision applied to all specific definitions related to the subject of energetic interaction. This principle also serves as a framework to study possible non-anticipated interactions between different types of energy.

The Analog Harmonic Resonance lays with elegance the foundations for all alternative healing systems. Becoming aware of its existence and becoming familiar with its mechanisms could lead to the most efficient combination of different types of energy for multiple uses.

Expand on this principle in particular, goes beyond the scope of this Reiki book. However, we deem it relevant at least to mention it, in the context of the comments about energy and its underlying mechanisms.

# LEVELS OF REIKI

For teaching, Reiki is structured by levels, allowing students to gradually get used to the technique, and to gradually understand the depth and spirit of this system.

Different Schools have different teaching structures and, in general, they vary from a minimum of three Levels to a maximum of thirteen. The Tibetan Usui System herein described is studied in Three Levels described below, plus Master to teach other people.

## Level I. Physical. The Awakening

At this level the student receives basic training to transmit Reiki energy. The personal cleansing process operates with some force at physical level, since biology is conditioned first to channel this energy.

No prior knowledge is required and the information transmitted has to do with the nature of Reiki, mode of action, application techniques and hand positioning. Main energy centers or chakras and Reiki Principles are also studied.

This level of Reiki is a genuine awakening since after receiving this first attunement a new univers is open to the student. .

## Level II. Emotional-Mental. The Transformation

A requirement for this level is to have taken the First level, however this does not indicate one level is superior to the other. Precedence is that it requires a work order with our bodies, so that the process be dosed and that the impact energy that is received can be absorbed without mishap.

The Reiki practitioner who decides to take this Level is aware of what he wants or needs to increase his Reiki energy potential. This level is also reached as a result of an inner need of transformation started in the first level.

Basic symbols of Reiki, which are energy attractors, are taught in this level. Reiki's usage techniques are enlarged and principles are deepened. Here emphasis is on emotional and mental bodies.

One of the most remarkable abilities at this level is the ability to send Reiki at a distance and through time. With this technique results obtained are equivalent to those hands-on treatments.

Few years ago, a minimum of Twenty-one days or a month were necessary to wait from Levels I and II attunements. Now and thanks to the significant increase in planet's frequency it is possible to follow Reiki's Level I and II on consecutive days, without compromising the quality of the results. Nevertheless, I have observed that attunements of Level I and II with a twenty-one day period in between permeate better into some people having more opportunities to arrogate this valuable tool.

## Level IIIA. Awareness. Fulfillment

This is a very special level. It is the level where Reiki Practitioner assumes a more clear personal commitment. The requirement is to be attuned in Level II and wait a minimum of 30 days to six month, depending on his or her level of practice.

It is also known as Inner Mastery since the student receives the master symbol, which significantly expands the intensity of the energy channeling and its scope.

Energy surgery is taught in this level as well as working with antahkarana mandalas and with crystal mandala, among other techniques. .

This level helps Reiki practitioner with his or her process of becoming a self-master. While the student may not initiate others, his energy and self-transformation potential are immense.

## Level IIIB. Mastery

Master Level is that in which the student learns how to initiate others in different Reiki Levels.

Like in other levels, personal commitment is the key to the whole process and the determinant of the results. It is important to highlight that being Reiki Master does not give the person the title of spiritual guide; what it means is that is capable to initiate others. Attunements received previously prepare the Reiki practitioner for the energy to flow in required amounts and quality so as to teach others.

Parallel to this, it is desirable that the Reiki practitioner can use Reiki for his own life process, which may favor him to reach higher levels of consciousness and, therefore can, in addition to starting with Reiki, support or stimulate other growth processes individual or group.

# LEVEL I
# The Awakening

# WHAT IS REIKI?

Reiki is a healing system working at a systemic level. It is essentially a balancing energy that facilitates the synchronization of the energy fields in all there.

This healing system uses harmonics of high frequency energy spectrum from spiritual planes, capable to align by resonance energy fields of lower frequency corresponding to the dense plane where physical, etheric, emotional and mental bodies exist.

The Reiki energy is inexhaustible and it is everywhere. It is available to all equally and it is initially transmitted hands-on, from one person to another. The person transmitting this type of energy is called Reiki channel or Reiki practitioner, getting this capacity by means of the attunement.

Reiki is actually a system of self-improvement. It is a path of spiritual evolution, of awareness raising and liberation. Besides the practical aspect of transmitting energy to generate resonance and balance, Reiki also proposes a philosophy of life, one way to explore ourselves and consciously confront this process so-called life.

History

There are several stories about the origin of Reiki which may seem more credible to one or the other. In this book I refrain from telling stories difficult to prove, focusing in other aspects of the technique that are of greater importance to the Reiki practitioner. Historic Information regarding Reiki can be found in an ample bibliography available in the market. .

What I can draw from common or notorious in the different stories is the following:

- There are registries of hands-on healing in Tibet since 6000 BC.

- There are Buddhist registries from 500 BC, year in which Reiki symbols to attract energy are found.

- In 1908 Japanese Mikao Usui (1865 - 1926) revives this ancient healing technique, reason why he is known as the one who rediscovers Reiki.

- It is said that Mikao Usui obtained much of the information about the symbols studying Tibetan and Buddhist manifestos, and how he was inspired from a non-human source, may be channeling during a 21-day meditation in Kurama Mountain, Japan.

- Mikao Usui recovered a millenary art.

- Mikao Usui started a healing lineage, transmitting to his students the initiation process. This is one of the most important aspects of Reiki which does not compare to anything done before. Many masters used hands-on healing but no system was left so common people could achieve the same. Therein lies the intrinsic value and the true magic of Reiki: Reiki System is for everyone.

• Hawayo Takata, initiated in Reiki by Chujiro Hayashi, direct pupil of Mikao Usui, was the vehicle for Reiki leaving Japan and becoming popular in the West.

## Schools

The first Reiki School is known as Traditional Usui Reiki and it is derived directly from Mikao Usui's teachings. Later various schools created by Masters expanding Reiki's vision have appeared, combining it with other healing systems or notions. In general, symbols are added, some extensions to the treatment's basic technique are made and the attuning is modified.

Many of these derivations are able to adapt the technique to improve acceptance or to potentiate their action.

Among the most important schools derived from Traditional Usui Reiki are:

Angelic RayKey (Reiki)
Ascension Reiki
Blue Star Reiki
Brahma Satya Reiki
Deepak Hardikar.
Dorje Reiki
EnerSense-Buddho
Gendai Reiki Ho
Ichi Sekai Reiki
Jinlap Maitri Reiki
Jo Reiki
Karuna Reiki
Karuna Ki
Komyo Reiki
Lightarian Reiki
Mahatma Reiki
Mari-El
Men Chho Reiki
New Life Reiki
Newlife Reiki-Seichim
Raku Kei Reiki
Reiki Plus

Seichim or Seichem or Sekhem     Satya Japanese Reiki
SEKHEM     Shakti Bija Mantra Reiki
Shambala Reiki     Sun Li Chung Reiki
Tara Reiki (Tara significa Kwan     Tera-Mai Reiki
Yin)
Tera-Mai Seichem     The Radiance Technique
Tibetan Reiki (Reiki Tibetano)     Tummo Rei Ki
Usui-Do (Tradicional Japonés)     Usui Shiki Ryoho
Usui/Tibetan Reiki     Vajra Reiki

## Symbology of Reiki

### Ideogram

The word Reiki corresponds to a Japanese ideogram expressing the depth of this healing system.

There are two versions of this ideogram, one old and one modern. Both are composed of two elements, one upper and one lower. The upper element responds to the phonetic Rei and the lower to the phonetic Ki.

This symbol has many levels of information that explain the energy work and philosophy of Reiki. We can find it in two variants:

### a. Ancient ideogram of Reiki

Even though this is not the oldest version, richness of its components allows a closest analysis of the concept and essence of Reiki.

To understand the meaning of Reiki we have to break down the symbol in its different elements Rei and Ki.

The Rei symbol, showed in the upper part of Figure 1, means "spirit not marked by its quality" or also "spiritual". This speaks of an implied meaning, something impossible of qualifying.

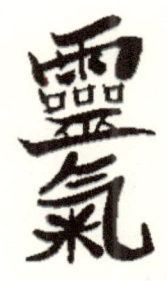

The Ki symbol, showed in the lower part of Figure 1, corresponds to the ideogram describing Qi or Chi in China; ie, this is the ideogram for energy.

**Figura 1**

From the union of the two symbols, there is a transcendental meaning, suggesting that Reiki is an energy that has not been classified, which nature is unknown, although it is known to be spiritual.

### b. The new version of the ideogram

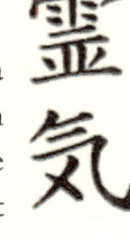

This second version was developed due to a spelling reform and does not allow too much research work in relation to the genesis of the word. Nevertheless, this symbol is also one right way to write Reiki

**Figura 2**

## *Color*

The colors associated with Reiki are violet and green.

During attunements people frequently talk about perceiving violet and green lights in a spiral movement. Amidst much diversity of possible manifestations during Reiki attunements, is notorious fin this similarity in more than 80% of attunements done by my person.

During Reiki treatment, it is likely to frequently perceive these colors. The same happens with people treated with Reiki.

Although to a lesser extent, approximately 3 out of 5 persons, also refer seeing this violet and green colors,

Analyzing the nature of these colors, we can see they represent healing and transmutation (green and violet respectively), which corresponds to the objective and action of Reiki. .

Green corresponds to Heart Chakra and violet to Crown chakra. Heart Chakra represents the energy of unconditional love and Crown Chakra represents the connection with higher planes. In this case colors could hint at loving and spiritual nature of Reiki. It also refers to a way in which Reiki is given: it is said that Reiki energy enters through the crown chakra of the Reiki practitioner and connecting with his or her heart chakra, from where it is distributed arms to the palms.

## What is NOT Reiki?

Reiki is neither a solution of all problems nor:

- A sect
- A religion
- Medication
- A refuge from the challenges of fate
- A substitute of our free will
- A substitute of our individual responsibility

These statements may make us doubt about the use of Reiki. To begin with, it is not a religious cult promising my salvation if complying with such and such precepts. My challenges of life will not be removed and I will continue making my own choices freely and being responsible for them. Moreover, it is not the panacea for each and every one of my physical ills. Then, what can I really get from Reiki?

The answer is: Everything. Even though it seems a contradiction it is not since the key is the intention of the Reiki practitioner and his or her constancy. Reiki is not going to dip you into a cult where all are treated equal and where your personal freedom is restricted and your choices of life questioned. In turn, it helps you to awaken your own power as human being. This approach is downright liberating.

If you practice and live Reiki, if you live, you're going to take life with greater balance, which will help you make better choices and feel more comfortable with your responsibility for yourself. Over time, you will see how the thread of your life is moving into other courses and much of what fate might have you in store disappears or turns into something different, more appropriate for your new level of consciousness.

The key is the integrity and intent of the Reiki practitioner with himself and his life. Reiki is an excellent ally, once you've decided to go your way.

No tool, technique, method, system or philosophy can replace human intention. It is the intention which is the real empowerment of people. Reiki is a wonderful bridge for you to lean out your true power, to your purest intentions, hand in hand with the highest part of yourself.

Intending Reiki has no limits, without intention Reiki is a missed opportunity.

## Advantages

Reiki Therapy, is presented today as one of the most attractive for the patient and the therapist, because:

- It is easy to learn.
- It is not invasive: no penetration of the body is required in any way.
- It is safe: causes no damage.
- It is easy to apply: does not require effort or special patient preparation. He needs only a little of your time.
- It is painless: Even usually has analgesic effect.
- It is modest: patient's intimate areas are not exposed.
- It is very effective: its beneficial action is well documented internationally.
- It can be combined with any other therapy without contraindications.
- It is applicable in any place or situation.
- The distance between the Reiki Practitioner and the patient, is not a limitation.

# REIKI PRINCIPLES

Dr. Usui developed the principles few years after creating the healing method. This makes Reiki a complete system for the improvement of the human being holistically, incorporating the conscious aspect throughout the process.

Usui was inspired by the five principles of the Meiji Emperor of Japan. The purpose is to show that healing the mind and emotions, through personal improvement, is an integral and necessary part in the Reiki's healing experience. The Usui system besides using Reiki energy must include the active commitment of the practitioner, as well as that of the patient with his own spiritual evolution. Reiki principles as they were written by Mikao Usui set out as follows:

*The secret art of inviting happiness*

*The miraculous medicine for all sicknesses*

*Just for today, don't get angry*

*Don't worry and be grateful*

*Work hard. Be kind to others*

*In the morning and at night, with hands held in prayer. Pray these words for your heart, and chant these words with your mouth.*

*The Usui Reiki method to change your mind and body for the better.*

*The Founder Mikao Usui.*

Today the principles are summarized as:

*Just for today:*

*Don't get angry,*

*Don't worry,*

*Be grateful,*

*Work honestly,*

*Show kindness to all living things.*

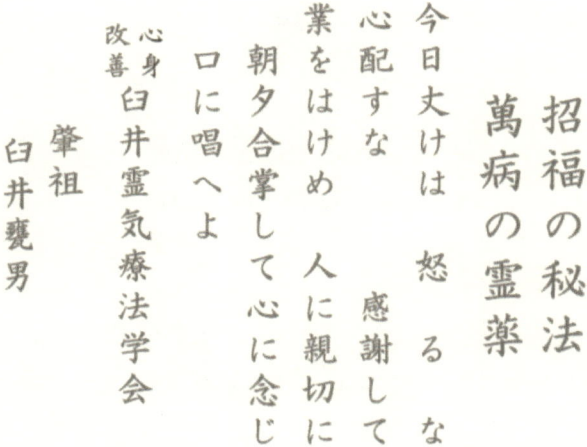

心身改善
臼井霊気療法学会

肇祖
臼井甕男

今日丈けは　怒るな
心配すな
業をはけめ　人に親切に
朝夕合掌して心に念じ
口に唱へよ

招福の秘法
萬病の霊薬

感謝して
なな

The original Reiki Ideals written by Dr. Mikao Usui

It is important to highlight that the Reiki practice should include the practice of the principles. A good way to become familiar with them and make them part of our lifestyle is: place them in a prominent place in our home and / or workplace and repeat every morning and every night in order to set these ideas in our mental and emotional bodies. In the section devoted to Level II will be discussed in more detail on the principles.

## Reiki Rules

- All people should ask for their treatment. This rule has to do with respecting the will of the people, their free will to decide when and how to be healed. It is also about respect for the Reiki technique.

- All treatment must be accompanied by an energetic exchange of some kind. The energy exchange is something that always happens, but in this case, the fact of requiring an exchange involves a major commitment of the person to heal and greater appreciation of the technique. What costs nothing is worth nothing.

The origin of these rules is frrom the experience of Dr. Usui in the early days of his practice as Reiki Practitioner.

It is said that Dr. Usui began to heal with Reiki most humble people, who in their majority lived on public charity. Over time, these people were to claim him because they had lost their livelihood, to be healthy because they did not get alms as before.

Facing this situation, Dr. Usui realized that he had to use Reiki to people who request it. Likewise, he warned that the treatment should be based on an exchange of energy, expressing the balance in the process of Reiki as well as the determination and will to heal from patients.

The Reiki practitioner should use his discretion as to these principles and treat them with open mind. Generally, intuition is an excellent guide for deciding whether to make unsolicited Reiki, especially in cases where people cannot decide for themselves. Intuition and common sense guide you in each case, whether it is appropriate to explicitly require an energetic exchange and the nature of the exchange. Please note that the money is the quintessential exchange energy on this plane, but not the only energy available to mediate this process.

## Healing

A note on healing. Many people are interested in Reiki, moved by the human feeling of helping others. In these cases, it may happen that the Reiki practitioner confuses his role in the healing process thinking that he is healing with his hands.

The reality is that we cannot heal anyone who has not decided to be healed. This leads to the conclusion that healing is a personal process that can only be done by one. No matter how many Reiki treatments a person receives, if she is not committed to her healing consciously or unconsciously, she will not get the desired result.

The Reiki practitioner or any other therapy should be very clear about this concept and never commit himself with the result of his work. The Reiki practitioner must channel the energy towards the patient. That is all his work and it must be flawless. But what the patient does with that energy is something that is beyond the scope of the therapist.

To try to ensure a better result, we can encourage the patient to express verbally his desire to heal. We know the impact of verbalization in creating the circumstances of life, therefore this resource makes the patient a little less patient and a little more conscious creator of his own process.

Avoiding compromise and responsibility with the result is a basic premise not to fall into two main dangers:

a) The belief that one is a powerful healer as patients respond well to treatment

b) Fall into sadness, frustration and distrust in Reiki when patients do not improve.

Be these comments worthy, not only for Reiki Practitioners, but for all therapists and facilitators of healing and healing processes.

# HOW TO CHANNEL REIKI ENERGY?

To channel Reiki energy it is necessary to go through an attunement that is primarily a healing process for the future practitioner of Reiki.

Often there is a discussion about the relevance of Reiki attunement as a requirement for channeling universal life energy. It argues that if this energy is universal and is there for everyone, no intermediaries are needed to get to it and use it. However, we know that is not enough for things to be there, available to all. Love has always been there and very few humans have been able to take and integrate it into their lives. The abundance of the universe is unlimited, but it is not sufficient requirement for every human being to feel it, live it, and experience it.

Under conditions of perfect balance of human beings, it is clear that access to Reiki energy is practically automatic. Under real conditions, the human is quite disconnected from its essence, unbalanced in several ways, which prevent contact with what has always been there for him. This is why attunements are a requirement in the vast majority of cases.

Besides attunements, theoretical training must be received about what is Reiki and how it operates, learn the working technique with the patient and of course, lots of practice.

## Who can channel Reiki Energy?

Reiki is a tool to be used by everyone. The energy does not judge but flows. Anyone can be attuned and transmit Reiki energy to others. Children are excellent channels because they are less contaminated by the consensus reality and block less energy.

Animals can also be initiated into Reiki and are excellent channels for this subtle energy. While a human being requires a tuning process for best results, the animals are automatically tuned and always will be moving vital energy.

Since the amount of vibration energy of humans is greater than animals, it is possible that the first are capable to move different qualities of Reiki energy.

There is an ethical issue of vital importance that must be emphasized here. No kind of moral or spiritual condition is required to get started in Reiki. You may be vibrating at a very low frequency, and yet, you can be initiated into Reiki. What can happen in these cases is that the initiate does not assimilate absolutely anything and does not connect with Reiki, or the initiate follows connection to Reiki and starts making transformations in your life.

That said, it is understood that the fact of being attuned in Reiki does not make you any better or worse than others.

However, the conscious practice of Reiki, it can stimulate and support growth processes important in the life of anyone.

## Process of Attunement

The process of Attunement consists of the opening of the chakras and that of central cannel, to allow passage of high vibrational energy and the creation of appropriate resonance. That is why during the attunement various reactions are observed such as emotion, joy, visions, colors, movement, drowsiness and more.

In general this process takes place in a private setting, to ensure there is peace and the minimum conditions of isolation from the outside. It is usually accompanied with music and ritual elements, according to the taste of the teacher and the type of Reiki in question. Candles, pictures of teachers, mandalas, essences, incense and more can be used as ritual elements.

The length of the process varies, depending on the amount of students, the level and type of Reiki. Some systems do several attunements for each level, while others make a single attunement for each level. The latter is the case of our Usui Tibetan Reiki. In this system, a single person attunement lasts approximately 10-15 minutes.

The initiation process is both a healing process. While preparing the student for the energy work old and new blocks are undone. This work is complemented by the self healing that the student must perform, known as energy cleansing.

All levels of Reiki require an attunement process and in all cases this process is complete only after 21 days Energy Cleansing.

## Energy Cleansing

The energy cleansing is essential to crystallize the healing process and therefore the attunement. This step is very important because matures the energy bodies of the student and stabilizes the attunement process. It requires some self-discipline and perseverance.

The energy cleansing is performed during a 21 consecutive day period and it requires that:

- The student does a complete self-Reiki treatment during 21 consecutive days.
- The student maintains a laidback lifestyle, no late nights, carrying a balanced pattern of sleep and rest.
- Does not consume liquor.
- Maintain a diet based on plenty of vegetables, fruits, grains and cereals if possible avoiding red meat[1].

During this process you may have some symptoms like dizziness, headaches, a gastrointestinal disorder, somnolence, among others. This is known as healing crisis and is usually of mild or brief symptomatic expressions related to the kind of balance that is being restored in the body. It is also very common to express unusual feelings and emotions during these 21 days.

Usually for Reiki self-treatment the best choice is at night, just before bedtime. During the first few days it is possible that the practitioner falls asleep. This should not be a surprise and the session also applies to the account of the 21 consecutive days.

---

[1] According to the latest research in nutrition, there are nutrition recommendations specific to the different blood groups and genotypes. It is very recommendable to follow those suggestions during 21 days.

After a while the contrary symptom may appear. It becomes more difficult to sleep when we do Reiki at night. In these cases we must move the hour of Reiki to the morning and take advantage of this energy load during the day.

If the sequence is interrupted for any reason, you must start again 21 days to properly seal initiation.

# REIKI SESSIONS

This chapter will present how to perform a Reiki session, what is necessary and most common types of sessions.

## General Conditions

Reiki can be done in public, in the middle of an emergency, without any requirement and no other support than its own intention, however this would be an extreme situation. In a more frequent situation where we can choose the time and place to prepare the conditions to work with Reiki, there is a group of desirable conditions that can facilitate and support the process. These conditions are:

- Choose a quiet, clean and airy place with minimal decoration and possibly without electrical appliances in excess.
- Create a type of work table or altar.
- Place on the altar incense or aroma diffuser, a candle, a plant element, some crystals and a glass of water with salt.

- The possibility to regulate the light of the place. Much clarity can affect relaxation; much darkness can hinder physical space management and patient.
- Preferably work on a massage table..
- Use soft music, preferably music with timestamps for the Reiki practitioner to be more focused on his work.

These recommendations should not be taken to the letter but as general guidelines to be applied using discernment in each case. You might find people who are allergic or just do not fancy the scents. In that case they should go without incense or other scent.

The general idea is to create an environment where the therapist and client feel at ease and comfortable; an environment where clients feel relaxed, safe and secure. Many times you should take time to listen and exchange ideas with the client before starting the treatment. This allows the person to release the tensions that bring from the street and create a more relaxed trusting atmosphere.

Achieving a relaxed atmosphere ensures that customers are going to be less defensive. This means that no discordant energies will have amplitude so large that opaque Reiki balancing frequency. Under these conditions the resonance can achieve large enough amplitude at the appropriate frequencies to dissipate the effect of discordant energies.

## Attracting the Energy

While the Reiki practitioner is capable to channel Reiki energy for life without any other accessory, it is important to support this process of channeling with the patient's intention and that of the Reiki practitioner.

## Intentionality

In the case of the patient, as mentioned above, it is highly desirable to make a strong, emotional, sincere and loud statement, which expresses its intention to heal this or that.

## Ken Yo Ku

The Reiki practitioner can use this simple ritual known as Ken Yo Ku that summarizes several important aspects for the successful development of the practice of Reiki. Ken Yo Ku is used to attract energy, ask for protection and help during the Reiki treatment.

The procedure is as follows:

1. Stand up, preferably in front of a window or space that faces outward.
2. Put your hands to the waist with palms up.
3. Move your right hand to the left shoulder and return to the previous position. Then bring the left hand to the right shoulder and return to the previous position.
4. Repeat the previous step.
5. Upload your arms forward at shoulder height with palms down.
6. Bring the right hand to the left shoulder to the hand pass without touching the left arm, as if he were clearing the aura. Repeat with the left hand and with the right again.
7. Raise both arms to the sky, palms up while legs slightly separated.

8. Make a call to the higher beings and Reiki master to protect, support and guide you.

9. Lower arms to the Namaste position, and say the word NAMASTE in greeting and respect to entities that accompany you.

Until step 6, a dry bathing or straightening the aura is performed, especially in the upper body and arms, which is where the energy will flow to be channeled.

Steps 6-9 are intended to ask for protection, assistance and guidance in the process. During steps 8 and 9 it is not necessary to speak loudly. Everything can be said mentally.

Ken Yo Ku can be done standing, sitting or lying.

## Heart Centered

Heart Centered is a fast way to invoke Reiki Energy. It can be done in any circumstance and can be equally effective if the intent was clearly and unequivocally expressed.

In cases of accidents, emergencies, irregular situations where you cannot run the Ken Yo Ku ritual, or simply as a routine method if you prefer, you can replace Ken Yo Ku by Heart Centering to attract Reiki energy.

To perform a heart-centered, bring hands to heart chakra (left below) and perform an invocation similar to that take place in step 8 of Ken Yo Ku. Complete with Namaste position, saying its mantra. As in the Ken Yo Ku, it is not necessary to say it out loud. Everything can be said mentally.

## Cosmic Wheel of Fire (CWF)

This is a valuable tool that serves to enhance the work of Reiki and also to support other processes in which some extra energy is needed.

This energy body is a gift from other planes, very useful for cleansing up our energy channels and chakras. It is also suitable for cleaning the aura and supports the process of correction of inverted polarity. La CWF has a centrifugal action to debug our fields. Also its high vibration can stimulate high frequency resonances, supporting our inclination to light.

This entity may be activated to support us in everyday situations such as rest or support therapeutic processes as the Reiki session. It is also useful for everyday personal issues like job interviews, performing a task and study.

Some aspects to consider when using the CWF are:

1.  The CWF has Higher Conscious. A high respect relationship is a must, first when invoking it and then when completing the process.
2.  The CWF must invoke from the I AM presence.
3.  By invoking this power give it a temporary framework for action. No power should remain indefinitely in any "place".
4.  You can take CWF where you consider that there is a blockage; it may act in any part of the body. It can be carried chakra to chakra to make a thorough cleaning of each one of them.
5.  You should always thank the CWF for the service given.
6.  It is recommended to activate it at least once a day and it may be used to sleep.

The CWF has a deep impact on you. Enter through the crown chakra and through the channels detecting and clearing blockages. At the end it will move back to one meter above your head waiting to be called back again.

## Test

One of the more subtle aspects of the techniques of Hands On Healing is the ability to detect energy blockages or irregularities using only hands. This method is known as scan.

There is no standard for this type of energy test. In general terms the basic technique is to put one hand about 5 inches above the patient, usually in the head, and begin to move the hand slowly throughout the body, paying special attention to the energy centers or chakras. Some people repeat the test by placing a hand to 10 inches from the patient's body to come into contact with the outer layers of the aura. There are experienced therapists who are comfortable working with both hands simultaneously.

During this process the practitioner will feel different sensory changes identified as temperature change, tingling, attraction, heaviness, increased density, among many others.

The interpretation of these signs should be made taking into account the data from the patient's cross-investigation. This subtle information is very useful for subsequent application of Reiki, because it identifies areas where greater dedication by the therapist may be needed. But in any way does not constitute a diagnosis to offer to the client.

## Exam with pendulum

The pendulum can be a useful tool when examining the energy centers of the patient. In this case it is important to take into account the basic principles of dowsing, among which is to ask permission, make a proper connection and properly formulate the question. The response of the pendulum shall be construed in accordance with the convention that has been established for this particular.

## Microcosmic Orbit

Deep breathing techniques, yoga, Qi Gong and many others, pay special attention to the use of the Hui Yin point to facilitate internal circulation of energy.

This point is located in the root chakra, more precisely in the perineum, the area between the genitals and anus. Contraction of this point allows the energy of the Microcosmic Orbit to rise up the spine to the mouth, following the route of the Governor Vessel meridian. This effect is enhanced if there is a simultaneous contraction of the lower abdomen.

To close the energy cycle of the microcosmic orbit, it must also support the tongue in the upper palate just behind the incisors. This position supports the process of energy flow, connecting the Governor Vessel meridian with the Conception Vessel meridian, which runs through the front of the body.

It is highly recommended that Reiki practitioners use this technique every time they start treatment or in the case of the Masters.

## A complete treatment with Reiki

This is the most commonly used method for applying Reiki, so we will begin the explanation from here. It assumes a properly conditioned place as aforesaid.

Both the patient and the Reiki practitioner should remove all kind of jewelry, metal parts and watches. In the latter, there is a possibility that the batteries are discharged.

The Reiki master should wash his hands before each session and be sure the patient has a minimum of repose. If the patient is very agitated or tense, first you should encourage him to release tension and relax a bit before taking a position on the massage table.

Also in this previous process, patient is helped to choose what he wants to heal. This idea of healing is then verbalize in step III.

The steps to follow during a Reiki session are:

I.   Perform Ken Yo Ku.

II.  Clean the place. With palms send Reiki energy in all directions of the room, especially to the corners.

III. Just before starting to work the patient is asked to verbalize his intention to heal. This is only done in cases where a communication allowing so is established.

IV.  Contract Hui Yin and close the microcosmic orbit.

V.   Bath the aura. With the palms of the hands 10 inches from the patient's body, made three clockwise ellipses over his aura, starting and ending at the head

VI.  Place the Reiki positions. 5 minutes for each position.

VII. Seal chakras giving a blow in the air on each.

VIII. Bath the aura again.

IX.  Release Hui Yin and open the microcosmic orbit.

X.  Separate from the patient. This is done mentally repeating the following: "I separate, I separate myself, I separate myself; from so and so I separate myself" and is accompanied by cutting and separation movements, which are carried out with both hands.

XI.  Carry out the Ken Yo Ku, this time giving thanks for the process to masters and beings of light that assisted.

After this process the practitioner must clean his hands, either by washing, shaking them strongly or passing them through the heat of the fire.

The patient may be asleep or being in a state of deep relaxation, so that should not be rudely awakened. This time is given to him to enjoy and assimilate the experience and then, very gently, guided to return to contact this physical dimension.

Usually is recommended a minimum of 5 sessions for each patient and in some cases a weekly follow-up session, according to the therapist. In chronic cases, 21 consecutive days treatment is recommended and later, weekly monitoring.

In some cases, according to the experience and intuition of the therapist, you can use selected positions instead of full treatment, either for lack of time or to focus on a particular anatomical or energy structure.

The long in one position may be extended beyond the recommended limit of 5 minutes, if the therapist feels so.

Self-Reiki

One of the main modes and the first a Reiki practitioner should learn is Self-Reiki or self-treatment. There are two basic types of Self-Reiki, a short and a long treatments.

The short form is to apply Reiki on chakras, taken in pairs, placing a hand on each. As in the case of the whole session, each position is maintained for 5 minutes. Some sequences may be (the numbers indicate the chakras 1. Root; 2. Umbilical; 3. Plexus Solar; 4. Heart; 5. Throat; 6. Brow; 7. Crown):

7-1; 6-2; 5-3; 4-4

4-4; 4-6; 3-6; 2-5; 1-7

The steps for this session are the same for a complete Reiki session, except for the IV and IX steps that are optional and step X, which is not done.

In long mode Self-Reiki, the Reiki practitioner will do on himself all positions as in a conventional Reiki session.

Grid

In this mode the work of healing is done among several Reiki practitioners on one patient at a time. The positions are distributed among the Reiki practitioners and one takes care of the patient's energy preparation. Regardless the latter, they all do the Ken Yo Ku at the beginning and end of treatment.

The grill is highly beneficial because Reiki energy is enhanced, i.e. the result is greater than the sum of the energies from participants.

Another advantage of this method is that it allows the healing process to run faster.

# OTHER USES OF REIKI

Since Reiki is energy and everything is energy, this high frequency resonance can impact everything that exists. There are no limits for Reiki energy. Limitations may exist in our minds, in our conditioning, but not in the energy. Some of the most used areas of Reiki are listed below.

## Reiki to food

It is known that food is one of the main elements of interaction of our biology with the environment. The nature of this interaction determines in many cases our state of physical, emotional and mental health. "We are what we eat" the old saying goes, so our food deserves the most attention.

The choice of food is becoming increasingly difficult due to the pace and style of contemporary life. Big part is eaten on the street and it is therefore very difficult to determine the origin or the raw material used in its manufacture. Actually, so does occur with food made at home.

A balancing element that can be used to compensate the Reiki practitioner possible damage from food, is to apply Reiki to the food before eating. By simply applying hands on the food bowl for a few seconds, the quality of food can be enhanced significantly and fully or partially override any harmful energy you may have.

The case of water is similar. Every time you drink a glass of water, take it in your hands for a few seconds and apply Reiki energy.

## Reiki to Plants

Plants receive with pleasure the Reiki energy. Reiki can revive plants that are virtually dry and have been given up as lost. This does not preclude proper attention to the care of the land, irrigation, nutrition, sun regime and other factors that can support plant recovery. However, in many cases the help of Reiki can be a decisive factor for the survival of the plant.

In the case of plants with pest problems, or nutritional deficiencies, it is possible to help with Reiki to strengthen their defenses and regain its healthy appearance, their brightness and color.

## Reiki to Animals

The animals are perhaps the most creative and receptive beings in Reiki treatments. They have enough receptivity to recognize and use Reiki energy in the amount and intensity appropriate for their healing processes.

Each species has its own characteristics, but in general all animals that have ever received Reiki, will look for Reiki whenever they need it. This means that if Reiki works with an animal, the next time they meet, it is likely that the animal looks for Reiki energy again, if need it. It will make all kinds of maneuvers until the Reiki practitioner's hands come in contact with his body.

A significant detail is that animals know where they need to be treated. Once they recognize that they are in the presence of Reiki, they will expose areas of their anatomy where the Reiki practitioner must put his hands. The length of each position is also variable and chosen by the animal itself. A treatment for an animal may vary from one to ten places and last from a few seconds to an hour or more.

What makes animals such good energy receptors, is that they do not have the powerful minds humans have and therefore are unable to lock themselves, or refuse to receive the benefits of energy as powerful as Reiki. Instinctively, they know when something is propitious and benefit from it with confidence and ease. Man interposes his mind, his reason and his ego, sometimes limiting the magical effects of this therapy.

## Chakra Balance

The chakra system of the human being, must work in harmony so that our bodies are balanced. First, the chakras should be the same size and proportionately spinning, each with the appropriate frequency.

The imbalance of the chakras brings different feelings of discomfort or uneasiness that may occur on the physical, emotional and mental level and can manifest as excitement or depression in one or more of these levels.

The Reiki practitioner can detect the state of the chakras by test or scan technique described above. In this regard it is important to make the comparison between chakras, remembering that balance is, in the first place, to compensate or reduce differences.

If we identify a down or blocked chakra, we can apply clockwise circular motion on the affected chakra. Then we can apply Reiki in the area for a minute or two to stimulate proper operation.

Then the a procedure is followed applying Reiki by pairs of chakras, so they are synchronized with each other. Different sequences can be used as:

4-4; 5-3; 6-2; 7-1

4-4; 4-6; 3-6; 2-5; 1-7

7-1; 6-2; 5-3; 4-4

After applying Reiki, hands are placed about 3.93 inches from the patient over the sixth chakra and after feeling its activity in our hands, we make a few clockwise turns. Then we put a hand on the third chakra and the other on second chakra repeating the above procedure. Then, fifth and fourth chakras, fifth and sixth and finally, the first and seventh chakras.

This process can be applied in conjunction with a chakra meditation. To apply this technique should also follow the procedure applied to the Reiki sessions.

# POSITIONS

The most common way to practice the energy transfer is by hands on the patient's body. Hands on does not necessarily mean that we will touch the patient's body. Depending on the person and the therapist, you can choose to have physical contact or not.

Some people may feel better treated if they feel the physical contact of the therapist; others prefer not to be touched by modesty or other reasons.

If you do not touch the patient is recommended to treat with hands between 1.97 and 3.94 off the body. In a channeling of Kryon entity, it is said that no physical contact method has a greater healing impact than using physical contact. My recommendation is to go with the intuition and treat each patient as circumstances demand.

Another aspect to take into consideration is regarding the front and back positions. Some Reiki practitioners apply first front positions and then back or vice versa. My personal recommendation is to apply either the front or back positions since, in most cases patients get deeply relaxed and even fell asleep. It would be counterproductive to wake them up or shake them from their state of relaxation to make them roll over in the massage table. Reiki energy acts at systemic level in our bodies, so that treating the front positions will also benefit any back imbalances and vice versa.

Under no circumstances hands should be placed strongly on the patient's body. This could affect treatment outcome..

## Front Positions

### POSITION 1

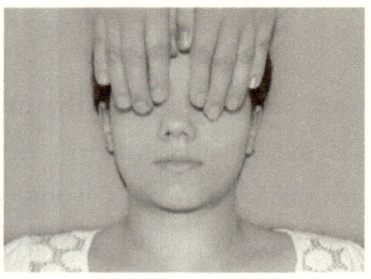

Hands are placed on eyes.

### POSITION 2

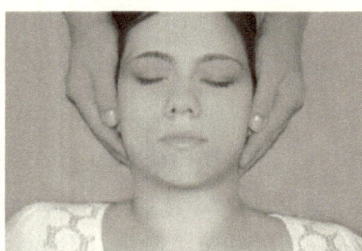

Hands are placed on the temples and ears.

## POSITION 3

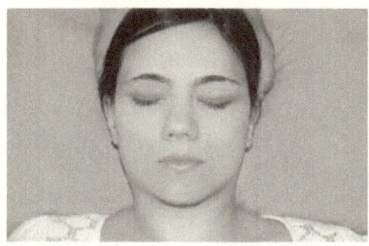

Hands are placed behind the head.

## POSITION 4

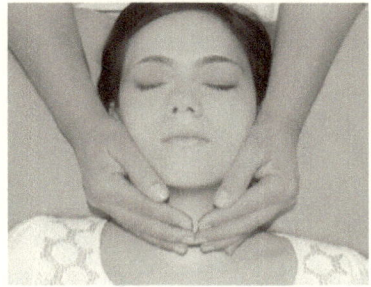

Hands are placed on throat or neck.

## POSICIÓN 5

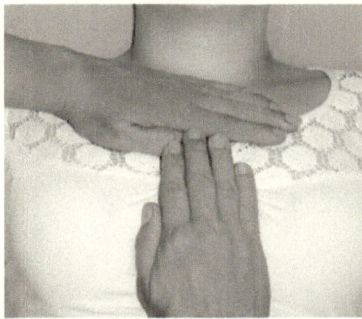

Hands are placed on chest.

## POSITION 6

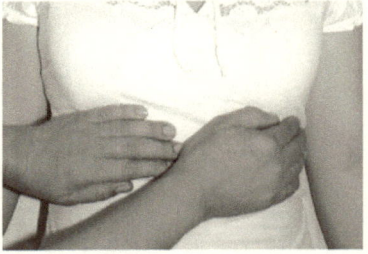

Hands are placed on the solar plexus.

## POSITION 7

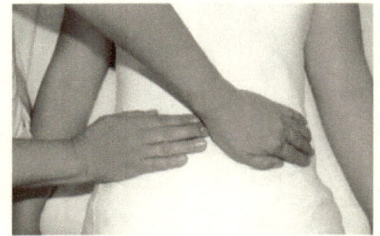

Hands are placed on the waist.

## POSITION 8

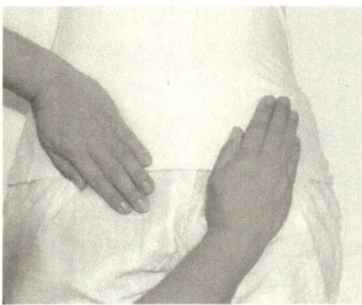

Hands are placed V-shape on the hips.

## POSITION 9

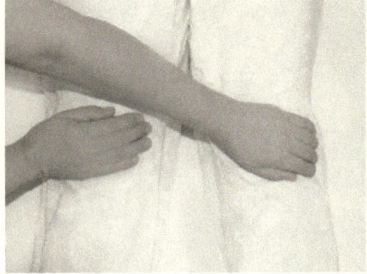

Hands are placed one on each knee.

## POSITION 10

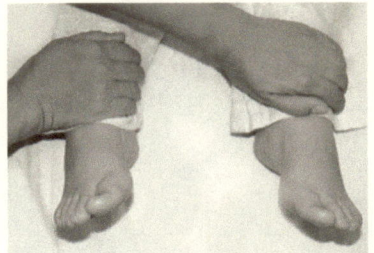

Hands are placed one on each ankle.

## POSITION 11

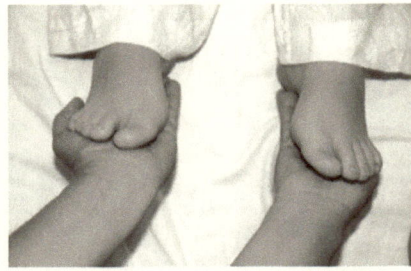

Hands are placed on the sole of each foot.

## Back Positions

### POSITION 1

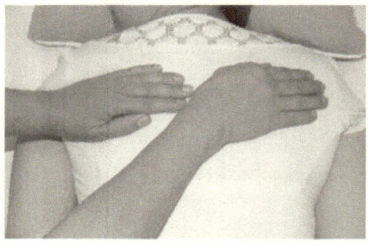

Hands are placed on the back, over the shoulder blades.

### POSITION 2

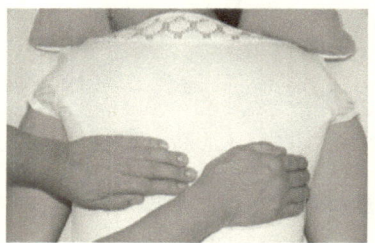

Hands are placed on the lower portion of the shoulder blades.

### POSITION 3

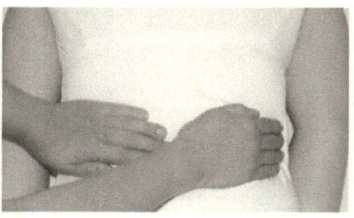

Hands are placed at kidneys level.

## POSITION 4

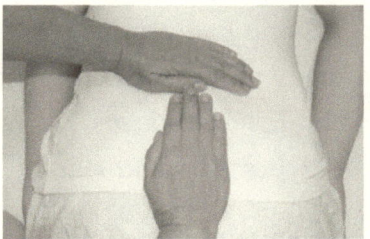

One hand is placed horizontally on the coccyx and the other
vertically between the buttocks, forming a T.

## Special Positions

### SPECIAL POSITION 1

Hands are placed on the clavicles, left and right of the neck.
It is useful for treating the bronchi. It relieves asthma,
bronchitis and cough. On an emotional level reduces feelings of
stress and anxiety.

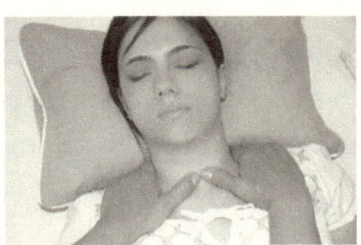

### SPECIAL POSITION 2

The hands are located right under the chest, to the waist. The
tips of the fingers are oriented toward the navel.

It is indicated for treating liver, gallbladder, pylorus and duodenum. It is recommended for all diseases of the liver and gallbladder, hepatitis, digestive disorders, flatulence, anorexia, spasm of the pylorus and hypertonia. If there are metabolic diseases detoxification is performed from this position.
At emotional level it relieves states of agitation and anger, depression and fear.

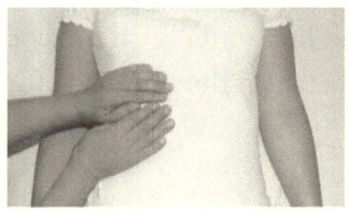

## SPECIAL POSITION 3

The hands are placed on the left side below the chest, the waist. The tips of the fingers are oriented toward the navel.
With this position, the objective is treating parts of the stomach and pancreas (insulin production and of enzymes), the spleen and parts of the large intestine and small intestine. It is useful for treating anemia, leukemia, the whole immune system, diabetes, infections, cancer, AIDS and celiac disease.
It strengthens the immune system in the case of diseases such as influenza, measles and mumps. On an emotional level can address the concern and obsessions.

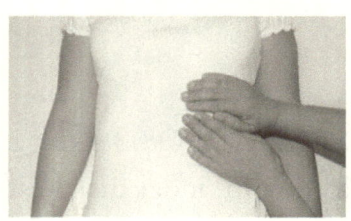

## SPECIAL POSITION 4

Hands are placed over the groin in a V. With this position you reach the root chakra and the sacral.

From here, the urogenital tract, intestines, appendix, uterus and bladder are treated. It is useful in diseases of the organs of the lower abdomen, circulation and digestion, as well as menopausal disorders. This position is further adopted for tumors of the breast, for his relationship with the female reproductive system. A mental and emotional level is used in neurosis of fear, sexual problems, weight problems, lack of drive, lack of prospects and pessimism. It stimulates positive thinking.

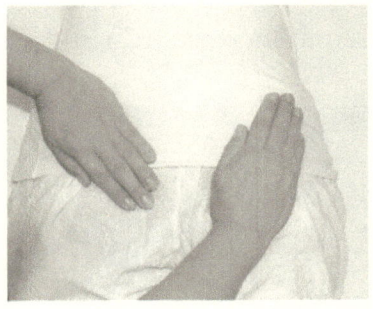

## SPECIAL POSITION 5

The person is lying face down; hands are placed on the back of knees.

In this case, a positive influence is obtained on the entire area of the knee. It is positive in cases of arthrosis, inflammation of the bursa and injuries caused by sports activities.

It helps to lose emotional blocks.

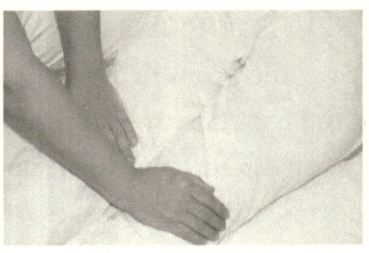

## SPECIAL POSITION 6

The person may be lying face down or face up. The hands are closed on ankles.

It is good to treat joint damage as well as diseases of the whole pelvic area. It is also used for arthritis, rheumatism and damage from the spine to the pelvic area; infections of the urinary tract. It is used to increase trust and stability.

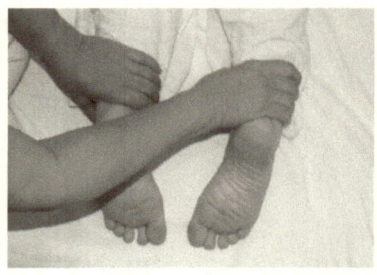

## SPECIAL POSITION 7

The person may be face down or face up; the hands rest on the sole of the foot

In this case every acupuncture points are achieved and activated. This position supports almost all other positions. This position should apply especially after a coma and after shock treatment.

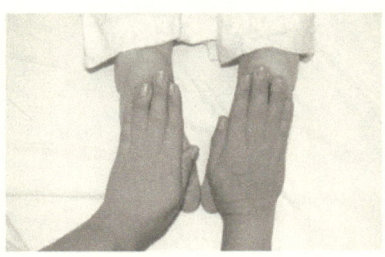

## SPECIAL POSITION 8

The person is lying face down. One hand rests on the sacrum and the other on the side of the foot where you feel pain. This is a special place for sciatic nerve treatment. The treatment should last at least 10 minutes.

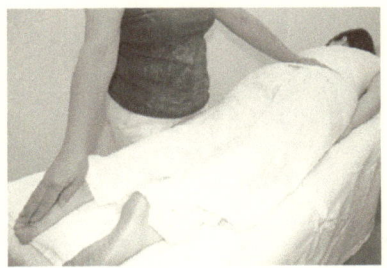

# LEVEL II
# The Transformation

# NECESSARY INTRODUCTION

To facilitate understanding of some of the material that will be at this level II of Reiki, it is necessary to introduce some notions that facilitate communication and understanding of the content. An analogy will be used to try to explain, at least partially, the concepts of time and space as could be seen from our Higher Self or from the higher dimensions or planes.

Imagine you are sitting in front of a huge lattice and that in every grid fits perfectly any of your fingers. The columns of the lattice, which run vertically, represent different times. The rows, which run horizontally, represent different points in space. By placing the fingers of your hand on different grids, you are contacting different points in space at different times.

Thus we come to the central theme of our analogy. Each of the fingers on the grids represents a human being, an ego, a personality embodied in a moment in time and a point in space, while the person sitting behind the lattice is the Higher Self of all these incarnations. A finger can be living in the time corresponding to the V century BC in Greece, what would make it a contemporary of Socrates, while another finger may be living in France on July 14, 1789 along with other Parisians marching to participate in the Bastille.

Each finger believes his time is now and the place is here, but this is just an illusion. Each finger has the feeling of being alone, of being independent and separate from the rest of the fingers, yet we know that this finger nourishes the blood and oxygen which nourishes all parts of the person behind the lattice; the same that nourishes other fingers. There is a vital breath that holds each finger belonging to a conscious being, the person; but that to the finger is almost unexplainable.

The Higher Self, the person behind the lattice, simultaneously experiences all that is happening with each finger in each grid of the lattice. All space is here and all times are now for this being. This view of space-time will facilitate intuitive understanding of how various healing techniques do operate.

# PRINCIPLES OF REIKI II

The principles of Reiki were outlined at Level I, discussing its importance to the Reiki practitioner and patient. Since this second level is related to the emotional and mental bodies, we will deepen a bit more on the content of these principles.

Reiki Level II not only extends the range and power of the energy transmission rate, but proposes the participant a more conscious integration and participation in the process of his own existence and spirituality. This level is that of the transformation, because the energy that is channeled will induce this process. If we support this transformation becoming aware of the principles and applying them to our daily lives, we can deeply impact our lives and change our reality.

Just for Today

There is only this moment, here and now. In the analogy above mentioned, a static view of "reality" was shown. Applying linear reasoning to explain the dynamics in this analogy, it would be understood that the fingers would move inexorably and steadily towards the column to the right, place where the next instant of time exists. This is because our view of time is linear and unidirectional. Eventually some fingers would move up or down, if the location in space during that fraction of time changes.

However, this linear view is part of the rules of what we believe to be, but nothing prevents the person behind the lattice, to move his fingers in a non-linear way and address a noncontiguous space and time. The idea is to show that this review is that the notion of linear time, of past and future is fundamentally illusory and belongs to the programming of our mind.

All I have is this present moment. Everything that can be done must be done at this time because there is no other time. Living in this moment tunes us with the Higher Self, who lives in total timelessness. It bears repeating that this is all you have and at this present are all the possibilities for all our incarnations. What we do now will impact all of our lives, for what is done all the time, impacts our Higher Self and resonates instantly to all that IS.

JUST FOR TODAY is a phrase often used in self-help groups such as Alcoholics Anonymous, to release any kind of addiction. The truth is that we should use it constantly, because our whole reality is an addiction. We are addicted to the memory, the conditioning, and the illusion of time and consensus reality. We are addicted to the duality and separation; we are addicted to inertia in life and we are addicted to death.

So, keeping the focus on the "just for today" can allow us to let go, drop the brakes and flow with the rhythm of life. If we have a purpose is the purpose we have TODAY and TODAY only. We should not postpone it, nor should we project it from the past, charging it with negative or limiting restrictions or experiences. We should not project it into the future, because the future does not exist.

## Don't Get Angry

Above all, few necessary definitions taken from Merriam-Webster:

> **anger** *noun. a strong feeling of displeasure and usually of antagonism. | | a strong feeling of being upset or annoyed because of something wrong or bad: the feeling that makes someone want to hurt other people, to shout, etc. : the feeling of being angry*
>
> **animus** *noun. : Basic attitude or governing spirit : DISPOSITION, INTENTION*
>
> *2: a usually prejudiced and often spiteful or malevolent ill will*
>
> *3: an inner masculine part of the female personality in the analytic psychology of C. G. Jung — compares ANIMA*

Anger corresponds to the activation of low-frequency energy in our emotional body, which creates an imbalance. Mostly it is an energy with ability to drag ourselves into unconsciousness, causing even reactions that are out of control.

Resonate with the energy of anger or rage, can cause endless problems in our organism. On the outside you can see how you delete all shadow of joy and love of someone's angry face. Often there is an excessive influx of blood to the head, which can cause stroke-like disorders. It increases heart rate and blood pressure increases as well, also increasing the risk of heart attack. Lot of adrenaline is released into the blood, which stimulates excessive body's metabolic processes, resulting in high energy consumption needlessly. The reason becomes clouded and things that are preferably not having said are said. While all this happens, the possibility of giving solution to the conflict does not go far, however it can go back. Anger is a sterile and harmful emotion.

Anger comes from fear and fear comes from ignorance. It also expresses loss of control or imbalance. The events unfold in a certain way and we cannot always be aware of the reasons for the occurrence of such a thing. But that is no reason to unleash the energy of anger. If we can understand that there is much more than what we see, smell and perceive with our senses, even much more than what we can gather with our intellect or imagine in our mind, we will be able not to judge but having an alternative to anger: acceptance.

The episodes of anger that arise in your life can be turn into an opportunity to be revised in you and so expand your worldview, that of people and things. Become aware of your reactions, be grateful of the ability to observe yourself and others and to have the opportunity to make the corrections you need in your life. If you get angry, do not feel guilty, just learn from it and get over it.

## Don't worry

Worry is a state of mind that is between the conscious and the unconscious, which is expressed notoriously on the conscious level and therefore is something that every person has the ability to manage with her intention and determination.

Let's see the meaning of the word worry, from Merriam-Webster Dictionary.

**Worry** *noun. a: mental distress or agitation resulting from concern usually for something impending or anticipated : ANXIETY*
  *b : an instance or occurrence of such distress or agitation*
  *2: a cause of worry: TROUBLE, DIFFICULTY*

Let's also observe the meaning of the verb "to worry", so as to have a better understanding:

**Worry** *tv:   to move, proceed, or progress by unceasing or difficult effort : STRUGGLE*
  *2. to afflict with mental distress or agitation : make anxious*
  *3. to feel or experience concern or anxiety*
  *4. to think about problems or fears : to feel or show fear and concern because you think that something bad has happened or could happen*

You can draw some conclusions at a glance about this word. First is a thought with emotional effects. Another interesting aspect to consider is that it is an anticipation, that is, it refers to something that does not exist, that has not happened. This indicates that the concern is primarily a prejudice, that is, a thought or anticipated judgment about a situation, person or thing.

In relation to the effects of the concern, the above definitions refer embarrassment and obfuscation of understanding. It uses the concept of insistence that, in other words, denotes the spatial and temporal omnipresence of the concern. And last, but perhaps one of the main connotations causing the anxiety and fear.

In short, worry could see as follows:

**Confuse and permanent thought establishing a prejudice[2] with respect to someone or something causing us fear or anxiety.**

This concept describes quite accurately the notion of concern is commonly used when people face conflict and unpleasant situations in life. It also fits well with the well-known concern for other people, relatives, friends, acquaintances or even strangers.

In Spanish, the word "PRE-OCUPACIÓN", according to the Dictionary,

*PRE is the Element that enters into the composition of different words to mean local or temporary antecedence, priority, appreciation or superiority in the extreme*

*OCCUPATION – Action and effect of occupy // Activity, work, employment or task in which time is spent.*

In this view, the concern is a state prior to the action, where nothing has been done. It is a state of paralysis, so the above concept could be enriched as follows:

**Confused thinking, paralyzing and permanent, establishing a prejudice about something or someone that causes fear or concern.**

In modern life there are a lot of situations that generate thought-feeling of worry. The reason for this is that we are used to seeing the world from a perspective of inferiority that causes

---

[2] prejudice noun. **a** (1) : preconceived judgment or opinion (2) : an adverse opinion or leaning formed without just grounds or before sufficient knowledge.

prejudice tv. to cause to have prejudice. To injure or damage by some judgment or action (as in a case of law) a menacing and unsettling feeling about the possible unfavorable outcome of any event.

That feeling is a habit acquired and transmitted from generation to generation. It is one of many learned behaviors that are usually taken as essentially human, inevitable, natural and even beneficial. Actually it is a trick of the mind; a trick that keeps us inactive while life continues its inexorable evolution.

Reiki stands that does not serve to surrender to the frustration, nor charge against abnormal factors. Do not worry does not mean becoming indifferent. It means that one does not echo the incident or event causing concern; it does not let trap by it.

Concerns are the result of the feeling of separation from the whole. Live each day to the best of your abilities and tackling one thing at a time, without fear or paralyzing before fear or difficulties, without despair to resolve all. Ask for earthly and divine help and remember something very important: Everything passes and that worrying you, will also pass!

## Be grateful

In first place we will quote the definition of gratitude from Merriam-Webster Dictionary:

> *gratitude* noun. *The state of being GRATEFUL : THANKFULNESS. a feeling of appreciation or thanks.*

Gratitude is one of the greatest tools for life. Gratitude is recognizing that everything that is given to us is valuable. A good question would be who or what to give thanks? The answer to this question is simple and short: to EVERYTHING.

According to the mystics, each episode of our lives has been carefully and meticulously planned by the Higher Selves of all actors. This includes the "victims", the "perpetrators" and all facilitators and support group.

Gratitude is offered for the honor of experiencing life, because everything is part of our own plan. It is not only to be grateful for the events that according to our ego / personality are favorable to us and deny or criticize those who are not. A broad and wise view appreciates EVERYTHING that happens to us equally.

All that exists comes from a divine source that many call God. All the objects we found our way, all our sensory experiences, emotional and mental, are imbued with the divine consciousness.

To sustain ourselves alive requires a lot of commitment, a lot of energy and love. The simple fact of having oxygen to breathe, to have a beautiful and varied reality to explore, to experiment and to create, encourages us to live in eternal gratitude. Getting up every morning is well worth a prayer of gratitude.

Everything is energy and there is nothing that is energy projected by chance. There is a good reason for everything and this reason is always based on the greater good. Things are not always what they seem to be and do not always have all the answers since whole picture of the game is unknown. As we increase our level of consciousness what is incomprehensible will become understandable and that inexplicable will make sense.

The way to interpret experiences is closely related to the vision you have about yourself. One, in partnership with the

Higher Self, is the architect of its own reality. There is no one to blame, or to turn to complain. In confusing situations it is more appropriate to be thankful for the opportunity to experience it and asking for clarity to solve it, as well as becoming aware of learning so not to repeat it.

Gratitude is closely related to self-esteem. Low self-esteem makes it impossible to acknowledge what you have and what you ARE. More than to be thankful for what you have is to be grateful for what you ARE: a portion of divinity as a human walking on Earth.

## Work honestly

This principle speaks to have in first place, an activity or occupation. From this we derive several interesting corners to explore.

First, the occupation with dedication. It is very important to have an activity to calm the mind through which it rests and help the body to balance. From this may arise, depending on the chosen art or craft, the practice of creativity. However, it is very necessary to have an activity that is related with you and occupy some of your time. It may be a job or a hobby, but something to occupy time and mind creatively should not miss.

Second, there is the vision of the work as a means of livelihood. Here this principle speaks of the importance of being self-sufficient or at least have a minimum of self-support. This approach allows maintaining self-preservation instinct and care alert enough to not to get hurt and not to rest or depend on others, if it can be help.

Third, and closely related to the above is the issue of honesty. This principle has found various translations as "Work honestly" or "Earn your living honestly" and has spread to the idea of living honestly.

> **honesty** *noun. a : fairness and straightforwardness of conduct the quality of being fair and truthful : the quality of being honest b : adherence to the facts : SINCERITY.*

Apparently this is to approach the issue with ethical overtones not think it is representative of the type of energy that is handled impartially in Reiki, but that it may be a consequence of the Japanese lifestyle, as related to the tradition.

There are some derivations of the word honesty and composure, decency, propriety, chastity, modesty, etc., which are rooted in cultural patterns variable from one region to another of the planet and extremely changeable in time. Such narrow focus that sometimes can become elitist, establishes a level of judgment and separation between people who do not congenial to the spirit of Reiki.

I think that apart from all this, at the bottom of this principle underlies the notion of service in relation to the mission of life. Every human is born with an innate ability or tendency to perform some activity. This can be said to be the passion of the individual. You may recognize that this passion has come when the person carries on business with joy, with genuine interest and does not shy away from dealing with work. It identifies so much with him that it is sometimes difficult to move him to another activity. Because in reality, there are few activities that would make him as happy as that he does with love.

To find this kind of activity, work or service in your life, can make the difference between having a happy life or a miserable life. Between working to survive or serving for pleasure; can you imagine a world where everyone were happy in his work?

## Show kindness to all people

This principle speaks first about love.

> **kind** *adj. 1 : having or showing a gentle nature and a desire to help others : wanting and liking to do good things and to bring happiness to others*
>
> *showing kindly interest and goodwill. // Lovable*

While it is expressed as "Be kind to people" others translate as "Show love and respect for all living things".

The meaning of kind that says lovable, I think exceptionally summarizes this principle. We must be worthy of being loved and the only way to accomplish this is loving.

Love is something very different from being in love, attachment and possession.

Love has nothing with doing; there is nothing to do for that love to be expressed. To love something or someone is to let this person BE, to fully develop and to be able to make his own choices in peace and freely, without any judgment.

Love is a state of balance between things that keeps them close enough to interact, nurture one another and capable to operate as a system. Also sufficiently far apart so as not to invade, nor collide, or destroyed each other; so not to lose their identity, freedom and contact with the environment.

In practical terms, this principle teaches us to be and let be, above all things..

# LEVELS OF CONSCIOUSNESS

The levels of consciousness are an exceptional contribution to humanity, made by the psychiatrist, Dr. David R. Hawkins PhD. For decades Dr. Hawkins has performed countless experiments to evaluate hundreds of thousands of subjects and achieved corroborate the existence of a measurable and quantifiable vibrational pattern related to human consciousness.

Hawkins's extensive research has shown that there are different levels of consciousness, which are nothing but vibration levels expressed in Hz, the same unit used to express, for example, electromagnetic energy. This crucial discovery establishes an unprecedented connection between the language of physics and the language of metaphysics.

As a result of this study, Dr. Hawkins was able to develop a range of levels of consciousness, which assigns a name to some of these levels and relates to its frequency in Hz, among other variables. The names of each level of consciousness are characteristic of emotions and states of the human being. See table on next page.

Thus, one could say that if we feel anger or rage, we are vibrating at a frequency of $10^{150}$ Hz In other words, we are increasing the frequency amplitude of $10^{150}$ Hz. No doubt that this is very enlightening and can make the difference between trying situations instinctively, with a great deal of emotion and unnecessary drama, or treat them from a conscious awareness with a more energetic approach and less passionate.

Continuing with the scale of the levels of consciousness, Dr. Hawkins found that if a person remains some time in states below Courage (10200 Hz), will be attracted to lower levels of consciousness, so called these levels of consciousness, low energy attractors. Conversely, if a person remains sometime in states above the Courage, will be attracted to higher levels of consciousness. This is the case of high energy attractors.

When analyzing the Reiki principles in light of the levels of consciousness, you can observe what follows:

• Don't get angry: Anger ($10^{150}$ Hz) corresponds to a low energy attractor.

• Don't worry: Preoccupation is between Grief ($10^{75}$ Hz) and Fear ($10^{100}$ Hz), low energy attractors.

• Be grateful: The basics of a true gratitude are the Acceptance ($10^{350}$ Hz), a high energy attractor.

• Work honestly: It requires of a vibration of Willingness ($10^{310}$ Hz), a high energy attractor.

• Show kindness to all people: It corresponds to the vibration of Love ($10^{500}$ Hz), a high energy attractor.

| Nivel de Consciencia | Frecuencia | Emoción |
|---|---|---|
| Enlightment | $10^{700}$ - $10^{1000}$ Hz | Indescribable |
| Peace | $10^{600}$ Hz | Bliss |
| Joy | $10^{540}$ Hz | Serenity |
| Love | $10^{500}$ Hz | Veneration |
| Reason | $10^{400}$ Hz | Understanding |
| Acceptance | $10^{350}$ Hz | Forgiveness |
| Willingness | $10^{310}$ Hz | Optimism |
| Neutralty | $10^{250}$ Hz | Trust |
| Courage | $10^{200}$ Hz | Consent |
| Pride | $10^{175}$ Hz | Contempt |
| Anger | $10^{150}$ Hz | Hate |
| Desire | $10^{125}$ Hz | Longing |
| Fear | $10^{100}$ Hz | Anxiety |
| Grief | $10^{75}$ Hz | Remorse |
| Apathy | $10^{50}$ Hz | Dispair |
| Guilt | $10^{30}$ Hz | Gilt |
| Shame | $10^{20}$ Hz | Humiliation |

**Consciousness levels, according to Dr. David R Hawkins.**

It is admirable the natural harmony existing among Reiki principles, set a little less than a century, and the levels of consciousness, which is one of the most revolutionary scientific developments of recent times in the field of human consciousness.

Seen from the point of view of Dr. Hawkins, the relevance of the principles of Reiki to raise our vibration as conscious beings can be confirmed, even numerically. The simple systematic verbalization, every morning and every night, from the principles of Reiki, favors the presence of high vibrations in our mental, emotional, etheric and physical bodies. These harmonious vibrations are able to transform our behavior and perception of all that is.

# REIKI SYMBOLS

The symbols are one of the most important traditions of teaching Reiki. It is said that its origin goes back to Tendai School of Japanese Tantric Buddhism, which has a rich symbolic and iconographic tradition. It is also said that Mikao Usui visualized these symbols at the end of a meditation for 21 days.

For several years the Reiki symbols were kept secret and were only transmitted from teacher to student orally. It was not possible for the student to write the symbols on paper and so to learn them later. From this derived the fact that some symbols, especially the most difficult to perform, went through changes over time.

At present the symbols of Reiki Level II can be found in manuals, books and web pages. Although initially there were fears that these symbols were incorrectly used, the experience of recent years has shown that there is no way to use them to harm. Another fear was that someone who knew the symbols started practicing Reiki without proper initiation, something that has been seen that it is totally impossible to do, because the tuning must be performed by a qualified teacher before the energy can flow properly through the practitioner.

At Level II three symbols are taught, which are intended to expand the action and effectiveness of Reiki. And these are:

- Cho Ku Rei: The Power
- Sei He Ki: The Light
- Hon Sha Ze Sho Nen: The Love

## Cho Ku Rei: The Power

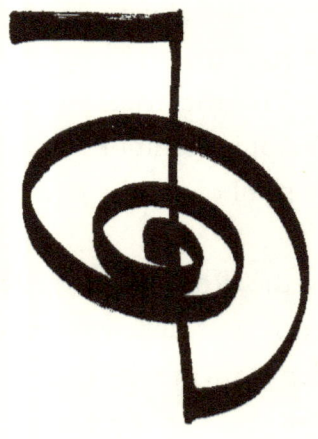

The name of this symbol in Japanese is Cho Ku Rei and it is interpreted as the symbol of Power or Strength

Action: *To Empower*

- Some of the meanings given to this symbol are: "God is here", "Universal Cosmic Energy here and now".

- Works primarily in the physical and to enhance the rest of the symbols. In general, it is used at the beginning and at the end of symbol string.
- Allows immediate connection to the Reiki energy, pulling it to the person or object of interest. It functions as a switch.
- It is the Protecting symbol par excellence.
- It is used to cleanse and purify the lower vibrational energies. This symbol transmutes energies from lower planes to higher levels.
- It does load high vibrational energies, and also allows excess energy balancing
- Allows energy balancing both in animals and plants and objects.

## Sei He Ki: The Light

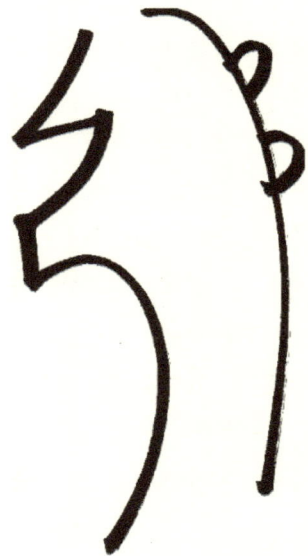

The of this symbol in Japanese is Sei He Ki and it is interpreted as the symbol of the Ligh.

Action: *Purify*.

- Some of the meanings of this symbol are: "God and Man are One", "The Key of the Universe".
- Works primarily at the emotional and mental level.
- Due to the form of dragon, it is said that this symbol spits out the fire of transmutation.
- Cleaning, cleansing, detoxification and disintegration of negative energies in people, animals, plants, objects and places.
- Reestablish emotional and mental balance.
- Works very well at subconscious level.

- For the cell-level reprogramming beliefs, karma, removal of votes, etc.
- Helps to develop the Cosmic Consciousness.

## Hon Sha Ze Sho Nen: The Love

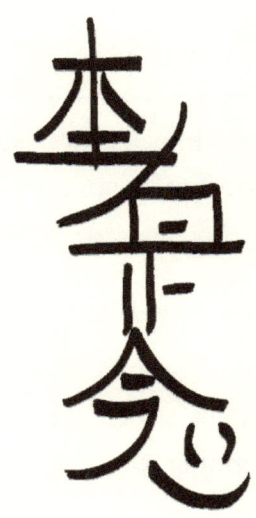

The name of this symbol in Japanese is Hon Sha Ze Sho Nen and it is interpreted as the symbol of Love.

Action: *Channel*

- Some of the meanings of this symbol are: "Neither past nor present nor future", "Distant Healing" y "Code of Absence".
- It is the most powerful symbol at this level. It works at a spiritual level.

- This healing symbol operates blurring the boundaries of space and time.
- Governs the mind, for connecting to the spiritual plane, brings order to the conscious mind.
- Acts on the conscious and the unconscious.
- One of its specific applications is recovery of mental health.
- Its application in distance treatments is as powerful as it is to place the hands directly on the patient.
- Another application is to support other people remotely, providing balance and harmony.
- Knowledge of past lives. It allows interacting with the Akashic Records.

These are the basic symbols shared by almost all Reiki systems, but there are many other symbols that are delivered to Reiki practitioner depending on the level and the system of Reiki that is studying.

## Personal Symbols

There are also other types of symbols that are called personal symbols. Sometimes the Reiki practitioners receive other symbols, either during initiation or during their practice as therapist. These symbols can be used in treatment or with any of the Reiki energy techniques used by the Reiki practitioner. It is very important to go with the intuition in these cases. It is said that when the Reiki practitioner becomes master, must include personal symbols in their initiations.

# REIKI II TREATMENT

## The use of the Symbols

To use the Reiki symbols, they are drawn in the air, directing them in the desired direction: a chakra, an anatomical region, a plant or any object or point of interest. Imaginarily, the symbol is pushed three times in the same direction, repeating with every gesture, its mantra or name in Japanese. Whenever you use a symbol, you must perform this same procedure.

If it is not appropriate to use your hands, you can draw the symbols and make the three thrusts mentally. Likewise, the mantra can be said loudly or mentally.

If a symbol is drawn wrong, you can delete it with your hand, making the gesture as if erasing on a blackboard and intention on the action. If the symbols are poorly drawn, which is very often the first few days, there is no cause for concern. We are not alone on this trip and the masters who accompany us know the intent and symbols can be corrected by us.

## *In which order are used*

General order of symbols is the following:

1. CKR – Cho Ku Rei
2. HSZSN – Hon Sha Ze Sho Nen
3. SHK – Sei He Ki
4. CKR – Cho Ku Rei

Some variations to this scheme could be:

- Eliminate CKR at the beginning. (HSZSN, SHK, CKR)
- Eliminate HSZSN if is not remote treatment and y one believes that SHK and CKR are enough. (CKR, SHK, CKR) (SHK, CKR)
- Eliminate SHK

There are many references in the literature which recommends what symbols to use with this or that disease. Personally, I think it's best to know what we are calling to each symbol and then used to dictate the intuition. If in doubt, I recommend using three symbols. We know they can not hurt and they can do much good.

Complete Reiki Treatment

As mentioned in Level I, this is the most widely used method for the application of Reiki. It assumes that the place is properly conditioned as discussed above.

Both the patient and the Reiki Practitioner should remove all kind of jewelry, metal parts and watches. As noted in the procedures of Level I.

The Reiki practitioner should wash his hands before each session and ensure that the patient has a minimum of calm. If the patient is very agitated or tense, first try to release some tension and relax a bit before taking a position on the massage table. If the mental and emotional bodies are excited, they will resist the harmonic vibration of Reiki, preventing for the proper resonance to occur.

Also in this previous process the patient is guided to choose what he wants to heal. This idea of healing is then verbalize in step V. The steps to follow during a Reiki session are:

I.     Perform Ken Yo Ku.

II.     Draw the appropriate symbols on hands. Ex HSZSN, SHK, CHR

III.     Apply on your own body the CKR symbol, from seventh chakra to the root chakra, as if it would be applied by another person.

IV.     Clean the place. With palms Reiki energy is sent in all directions of the room, especially at the corners.

V.     Just before starting to work with the patient he is asked to verbalize his intention to heal.

VI.     Contract Hui Yin and close the microcosmic orbit (See Level I).

VII.     Bath the aura. With the palms of the hands to 10 inches from the patient's body, made three clockwise ellipses on his aura, starting and ending at the head.

VIII.     Apply to the patient the appropriate symbols on the crown chakra; on the front, from the

6th to the root chakra and the soles of his feet. You can only use CKR, or SHK and CKR, or the sequence HSZSN, SHK, CHR. This to be a choice of the Reiki practitioner.

IX. Place Reiki positions. Three minutes per position are enough. If more or less time is needed go with intuition.

X. Seal chakras giving a blow in the air over each chakra.

XI. Repeat step VIII.

XII. Repeat step VII.

XIII. Release Hui Yin and open microcosmic orbit (See Level I).

XIV. Separate from the patient. This is done mentally repeating the following: "I separate, I separate myself, I separate myself; from so and so I separate myself" and is accompanied by cutting and separation movements, which are carried out with both hands.

XV. Carry out the Ken Yo Ku, this time giving thanks for the process to masters and beings of light that assisted.

After this process the practitioner must clean his hands, either by washing, strongly shaking or passing them through the heat of the fire. Follow the rest of the recommendations of Level I.

Self-Reiki

After initiation of Level II, the Reiki practitioner must perform again an energy cleansing process for 21 days, as described in Level I. In this case, the same rules apply to self-Reiki indicated in Level I, but this time following the sequence of steps for Level II which includes the use of symbols.

The above sequence applies to the whole session, except for steps VI and XIII and XIV that are optional.

Grid

With Level II, the grid is enriched by the use of symbols. In this case, all involved Reiki practitioners work with symbols for themselves, on their hands and body, as shown in steps II and III of the full treatment of this level.

Only one of the Reiki practitioners will bath the aura and draw the symbols on the patient, as indicated in Steps VII, VIII, XI and XII of the entire treatment.

The duration of positions at Level II is 3 minutes. Also, the healing potential of energy is much higher. The fact of working with symbols notoriously expands the impact of Reiki in patients.

Distant Reiki

This is the most powerful and most revealing learning that takes place at this level. For Distant Reiki is always used HSZSN symbol. This symbol has the ability to connect with Unconditional Love.

In terms of the analogy presented at the beginning of this level, HSZSN allows acting from the perspective of the connection with our Higher Self, i.e. the person sitting behind the grid. From this position, there is no point of time or point in space that cannot be healed.

Distant Reiki allows sending energy to people, animals, plants, objects and situations at any place and time. You can send energy over time, both the past and the future. If you think HSZSN allows Reiki energy to move from the perspective of the person behind the dash, all the events of the past and the future are accessible from this point.

For the past, Reiki energy can be used to balance, heal or reevaluate previous events. Here you can change the old way events are interpreted in the present. You can send Reiki to a difficult relationship in the past, so that the perception of the people involved is expanded and having more loving impressions and reactions.

A very desirable requirement in the case of sending Distant Reiki to people is that they know that they will receive this energy and so be ready. The reason for this is that many times, when sending Distant Reiki, patients have referred sensations and symptoms that if present when at work environment or requiring certain levels of attention, can cause unwanted interference.

You can use several ways to apply Distant Reiki, at this point the creativity has no limits, but all of them involve the use of witnesses.

## Witnesses

Witnesses are nothing but means to represent a subject or object that you want to work energetically. Just as you need a phone number to call someone or an address to send an email, in the work with energy a way to identify the recipient of the energy is necessary. Such identification is performed through witnesses. When applying energy to a witness, we are expressing our intention to send that energy to the object or subject represented by this.

There are different types of witnesses. Among the most important we have the following:

Biological Witnesses: Biological element is any person, animal or plant to be treated. It could be a portion of hair, hairs, nails, blood, leaves, roots, feathers.

Impregnated Witness: It consists of a garment or object used, impregnated by the energy of the person or object of the place you want to heal.

Picture Witness: A photo of the subject (person, animal, plant, location) of treatment is an excellent way to facilitate sending Reiki energy. In this type of witness radiographs and photocopies of documents are included, among others.

Made-up Witness: Is to write down on paper the data identifying the subject (person, animal, plant, location) of treatment such as name, date of birth, city.

Mental Witness: The mental image of a subject (person, animal, plant, location) of treatment is sufficient to send Reiki energy. It is commonly used with subjects familiar to the therapist. Information can also be used to bring in a witness mental image produced as the subject, ie, a mental image data name, location, etc. is created.

Model Witness: It is an object used as means representing the subject being treated. As an example, a stuffed animal, a pillow or the Reiki practitioner's thigh, can be used.

Steps

There are two fundamental modalities of Distant Reilki :

- Complete Distant Reiki with every position as if you were on the premises. In this case we use the witness Model or perhaps the witness photo, when having a full body picture of the patient.
- Short Distant Reiki applying energy to the patient as a whole, for a minimum of 6 minutes. In this case we usually work mostly with photo, mental and manufactured witnesses.

The steps to follow during a Distant Reiki session are:

I.  Perform Ken Yo Ku.

II.  Draw on hands the symbols HSZSN, SHK, CHR

III.  Apply on your own body the CKR symbol, from seventh chakra to the root chakra, as if it would be applied by another person.

IV.  With hands in Namaste, make a mental connection with the Higher Self of the patient indicating session is going to start. Be alert to any indication that would be received for not following the treatment.

V.  Contract Hui Yin and close the microcosmic orbit (See Level I).

VI.  Bath the aura. With the palms of the hands on the used witness, with three clockwise ellipses.

VII.  Apply to the witness the appropriate symbols; once is it is Short Distant Reiki or; on the crown chakra; on the front and the soles of its feet when Complete Distant Reiki. You can only use CKR, or SHK and CKR, or the sequence HSZSN, SHK, CHR.

VIII. Place Reiki positions on the witness for three minutes per position, in the case of Complete Distant Reiki. Place Picture/Manufactured witness or visualize mental image on the hands during a minimum of 6 minutes, when doing a Short Distant Reiki treatment.

IX. After completing the positions, call the Higher Self of the person to inform it the session had completed and send the symbols three times with hands to the patient or the situation

X. In case of Complete Distant Reiki seal chakras giving a blow in the air over each chakra.

XI. Repeat step VII.

XII. Repeat step VI.

XIII. Release Hui Yin and open microcosmic orbit (See Level I).

XIV. Separate from the patient. This is done mentally repeating the following: "I separate, I separate myself, I separate myself; from so and so I separate myself" and is accompanied by cutting and separation movements, which are carried out with both hands.

XV. Carry out the Ken Yo Ku, this time giving thanks for the process to masters and beings of light that assisted.

To work with the Model witness, it is necessary to associate the witness with the object or subject to whom Reiki is being sent. This is accomplished by placing the symbols HSZSN and CKR on the witness and then repeating three times the name of the object or subject of treatment while patting on the Model witness.

# OTHER APPLICATIONS OF SYMBOLS

## Mental Programming

This technique allows programming work beliefs, using phrases or statements. The phrase may select the therapist or the client, but it should be something that the latter feel fully committed.

Phrases like: "I'm rich and prosperous", "I am who I am", "My Time Is Perfect", "Joy of Health and Happiness", "My Life is Love", "I am Light" can be used

### *Steps*

I.   Perform Heart Centering.
II.  Bath the aura.
III. Apply CKR in the crown chakra and in feet.
IV.  Repeat three times the name of the person.
V.   Apply SHK in the crown chakra.
VI.  Repeat chosen affirmation.

VII. Place the no dominant hand on the forehead and dominant under the occipital. Hold this position for 3 minutes while mentally repeating the affirmation.

VIII. Remove your hand from the forehead and apply Reiki for 3 minutes in the occipital region, without repeating the affirmation.

The client must repeat the affirmation mentally while performing therapy. This technique can also be used to self mental programming.

## Some Useful Ideas

### *Protect Housing*

Apply CKR whenever we go out or enter the house. CKR also be applied in the six directions of the house: north, south, east, west, up and down.

If mental and emotional loads, we recommend using the SHK. You can also use HSZSN in case you need to handle conflicts related to past or karmic aspects.

### *Protect yourself and others*

We trace the CKR around the body: on the sides, the front, and back and on the root chakra. Whenever you go out of the house CKR can be applied at least at the front. It can be applied to any other person.

As in the previous case, SHK can be used for emotional / mental protection. If the situation is to prepare in advance for a business meeting or an important meeting, you can use the HSZSN with other symbols.

## Emergency Support

There are emergency situations such as a car accident or a fall, which looks certain degree of imbalance or have the potential to attract lower vibrations. In these cases you can send CKR by hand or mentally, bearing in mind the intention of the symbol: "God is here" or "Universal Cosmic Energy here and now". In this way you are injecting high vibration energy to the situation or person concerned, facilitating the harmonization of the ongoing process or event.

## Water and Food

CKR may be applied to everything we eat, to reduce the potential harmful effects or toxic. Apply the symbol on the food and placing the hands on the plate for a few seconds, helps balance the food energy.

If you consume any medication, you should apply the symbols just before eating.

Water should also be treated and impregnated with the energy and the Reiki symbols to help us attune. Through Masaru Emoto's experiments with water, we can understand the benefits it can bring in to our lives.

## The Notebook Technique

It is helpful to use a notebook to record the goals to be achieved. This technique is preferably used to process personal goals.

In the reverse of cover and back cover, draw the symbols with their names written three times. If desired, cover them with a photo or paper not to be seen with the naked eye.

Then goals are written in the book and a minimum of three minutes of Reiki is applied to each book cover. Then Reiki is applied every day for at least 3 minutes, taking the notebook between the two hands.

To clarify petitions drawings can be made, paste pictures in the notebook, coloring to highlight something, in short, be creative! The limit is set only by oneself.

## The technique of the box

You take a box which will have the Reiki symbols with their mantras repeated three times, written in the bottom of it. In this box you can place multiple requests such as ongoing healing treatments , third-party healing requests, group goals and any requirement with little data.

Following a minimum of six minutes of Reiki is applied to the box. Reiki is then applied every day for at least 3 minutes, taking the box between the two hands.

It's recommended that you have a notebook to record the results obtained with the technique of the Notebook and of the Box. This will increase your confidence in these techniques which is nothing else but your trust in your connection to your own Higher Self.

# ADDITIONAL INFORMATION

This chapter is to present information I received during two sessions of Reiki. One is about what happens in a Reiki treatment and the other about hand positions.

In both cases, the information was transmitted by clients with certain levels of ESP, immediately upon completion of the session. I allow myself to share these experiences with the reader to expand their vision of what this practice can mean. In no way these visions are established as "truth", but as information that can favor understanding of Reiki.

## What does happen in a Reiki session?

This story took place in a grid type session, where I am accompanied by another Reiki master. During the Reiki treatment the patient, who is a natural clairvoyant, could see a beam of light-energy-entering my head and the other teacher. These beams were bright white light in its center and towards the periphery it was turning into a rainbow.

The beams were very wide up and were gradually reduced as it descended to fit perfectly into the crown chakra

This light came into our hearts and from there went to the hands. From the palms a multicolor beam came out and from the finger rays out as fine lines of light of different colors. Both the beam as the lines could reach a length of two feet.

She also observed a column of bright, intense light as a cylinder, beside each Reiki practitioner. She identified this energy as Reiki masters from other planes that assisted us during the Reiki treatment.

On a personal level, she felt a very subtle energy that ran through her bodies, cleaning and balancing everything in its path. In the etheric body she felt a powerful cleaning effect and compared it to shake and deep cleaning a carpet.

## Positions of hands

On another occasion, after applying Reiki to a patient who has the gift of clairaudience, after coming out form a deep relaxation she stared at me and then said:

"Teachers told me to give you this information about the positions of the upper part of the body.

The first position is to eliminate unnecessary thoughts and clear your mind.

The second is to increase understanding. It improves the ability to interpret the real meaning behind the words and deeds.

The third position is to clean the subconscious of unnecessary information. It completely sweeps it, releasing very deeply hidden constraints, unfulfilled desires and much more.

The fourth is to learn to communicate, to say clearly what is meant. It also has to do with the opportunity in terms of: What to say and when to say.

Finally the fifth position seals all the previous work. "

In my practice with clients and also in my personal capacity Self-Reiki sessions, I have intuitively verify the appropriateness of this information.

# LEVEL III
## The Realization

# INTRODUCTION TO LEVEL III

The Level III of Usui Tibetan Reiki system significantly increases the vibratory capacity of our energy bodies and constitutes personal mastery. It is a great responsibility level for the Reiki practitioner, where there are techniques that require more individual work and deep conviction and dedication to properly facilitate the healing process. The work is more subtle.

The work is from the heart level, developing self-confidence and attracting our attention increasingly to our Inner Master, to be our true and eternal being. Our intuition and our capacity to deal with peace and harmony in everyday situations are also amply enhanced.

You learn a new symbol that is the Traditional Usui master symbol. This symbol expands the power of channeling Reiki energy. It is also an element that enhances the connection between the physical and the spiritual planes.

Antahkarana Tibetan mandalas are introduced. These expand and enhance the use of Reiki, both personally and in working with others and with the planet.

The Reiki practitioner will be attuned en various procedures in this level that will be of help in his practice, allowing him to perform deeper intervention in facilitating the process of healing. Among which are the re-polarization, energy surgery and return home.

## Lineage

Reiki is a discipline that is taught from master to disciple. Unlike other techniques that are taught in schools, colleges and universities, many of which can be learned through self, Reiki requires that a teacher will be present to personally do the attunement. There is not headquarters to endorse or certify a Reiki practitioner, so the best way to "certify", "execute" or "validate" your skill is by exposing the source of your knowledge. This is done through a Reiki lineage.

The lineage also serves to honor masters who came before us and made the miracle of Reiki possible for us. What follows is my lineage, your lineage if you choose, with deep respect and gratitude to all the masters who I quote. I also extend my respect and gratitude to all masters in light of all times, for sustaining the miracles on earth.

The new initiate inherits the lineage of his master, as if it were a genealogy of Reiki. It is important to note that under no circumstances lineage is an expression of the quality, completeness, efficacy or a Reiki degree of authenticity. No matter how far or near the initiate is from Dr. Mikao Usui, his entitlement to channel Reiki is as valid as that of the founder himself.

Rather than searching for a place in the lineage bringing him closer to the master Mikao Usui, the initiate must find within himself the strength and integrity necessary for living and practicing Reiki according to the principles of this discipline, following and sticking to their own Inner Master.

## *My Reiki Lineage*

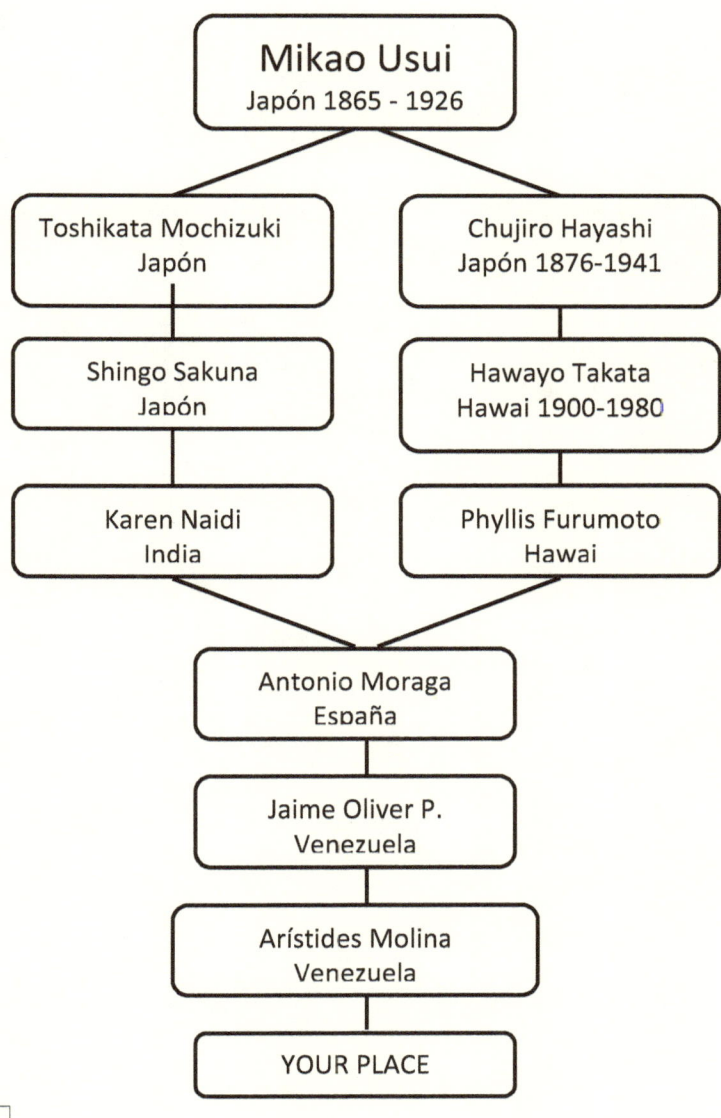

# SYMBOLS OF LEVEL III

## Dai Ko Myo: Master Symbol

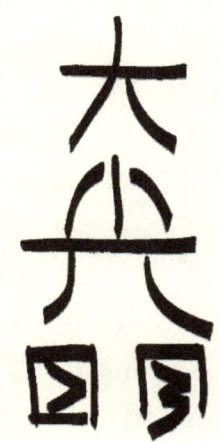

Tibetan Dai Ko Myo

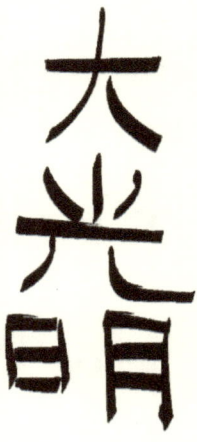

Japanese Dai Ko Myo

The name of this symbol in Japanese is Dai Ko Myo and it is interpreted as the Master symbol.

Action: Connecting Physical Self with Higher Self.

- Some meanings are: "Great Bright Light", "Great Being of the Universe shines on me", "House of the Treasure of the Great Radiant Light", "The Cure of the Soul".
- As in the case of HSZSN, there are different versions of this symbol. Those that will be used in this course are those illustrated above, corresponding to the Female Dai Ko Myo or Tibetan and Male Dai Ko Myo or Japanese, respectively.
- The primary use of the Dai Ko Myo (DKM) is to make Reiki initiation. As a Master symbol it encapsulates the phenomenon Reiki itself.

- DKM contains summarized and enhanced energy of the three Level II symbols.
- DKM is used to connect with your life purpose and it is used in all the work of protection and healing.
- Dai Ko Myo has a vibration higher than the Cho Ku Rei and therefore has a higher potential for healing and personal transformation.
- It is also used for unlimited power manifest in the physical world and is therefore the divine in physical form. It is said that "miracles" happen with this symbol.
- DKM can be used as a focus of meditation (can be used as any of the other three symbols).
- Recommendation is to be used in all Reiki treatments.
- DAI means great; great man.
- KO means light; fire taken by a man.
- MYO means brightness; the sun and the moon.

## Uses of DKM

It is used in all the activities that have been studied in previous levels of Reiki. This is used to call an energy that moves in a higher vibrational level all previous ones symbols.

To use DKM in Reiki sessions, you must use the same steps that were studied in Level II, using the DKM at the beginning of all sequences of symbols, especially at the following times:

- When drawing the symbols in our hands.
- When drawing the symbols on the client before the treatment
- When drawing the symbols after sealing the chakras.

The same goes for the grid, remote sessions, self-Reiki sessions and mental programming.

This symbol should be incorporated as means of protection for people and places, also add to notebook and box techniques studied in Level II.

The DKM symbol can replace CKR and SHK symbols, but not HSZSN which is essential for sending Reiki at a distance. The Reiki practitioner may choose to use only DKM when recommending the use of CKR and SHK, or DKM can be added wherever CKR and / or SHK symbols are recommend using.

Finally, DKM is used in all initiations of Reiki and in the procedures described in this level such as Surgery, Re-polarization and Return to Home.

# ANTHAKARANA

According to widespread teaching in Reiki, Antahkarana is a Tibetan mandala used to strengthen the work with this energy. Several authors handle different concepts of Antahkarana. However, I choose to transmit the related concept with the tattvas of Hindu philosophy.

In my research, I have confirmed that the word Antahkarana appoints the psychic organ and is at a high level of vibration, but still belongs to the world of limitations. To better illustrate what this concept of Antahkarana means, a subset of the category hierarchy of being or tattvas is present, in the following table.

According to this model, Antakarana or Antahkarana, is the expression of three of the categories of being known as Buddhi, Ahankaara and Manas. We could correlate to the words Intellect, Ego and Mind, respectively. According to the order of the tattvas, before Antahkarana there is Purusha and Prakriti, which are Shiva and Shakti covered with the veil of Maya and subject to the limitations of time, space, the will, knowledge and action. This contraction of the greatness of Shiva and Shakti - "male and female" principles prior to manifested existence-, forms the basis of the finite, the basis for subsequent separation.

| | | |
|---|---|---|
| 12. Purusa | It's Shiva after suffering Maayaa veil and the five Wraps of Ignorance. Despite such self-imposed limitation, Shiva is nevertheless the same. This Purusha is the inner Self in all beings. | |
| 13. Prakriti | Prakriti is a state in which the powers of Knowledge, Will and Action remain completely balanced, after suffering another contraction. Purusa, which is Shiva himself, beholds His Shakti, who is now listed as Prakriti, balancing the three branches. Shiva changed his views and began to be considered as an individual soul. | |
| 14. Buddhi o Mahát | It is the first manifestation of Prakriti. Buddhi is the determinative faculty by which you decide a course of action in your life. In sum, Buddhi is "the Intellect". Buddhi is also the principle that allows you to catalog abstractly some object, animal or person under a defined category. For example, "This is a dog", "This is a hat." | ANTAHKARANA Inner (psychic) organ |
| 15. Ahankaara o Asmitaa | It is the second manifestation of Prakriti. Ahankaara is the limited "sense of self". In sum, Ahankaara is "Ego". Its main characteristic is "self-ownership." Associates the "I" pure, which is a mere witness, with particular action or concept. For example, "I do my work", "I build buildings", "I love you", "I am poor", etc.  If you remove the Ahankaara the prayers would be as follows: "The work is being done", "The buildings are being built", "There's love for you", "There is poverty", etc.. Ahankaara also gives "volume" to everything. It is the cause for this 3D universe. | |
| 16. Manas | It is the third manifestation of Prakriti. Manas is a network of thoughts. In sum, Manas is the "ordinary mind" that is the source and the controller of future Perception and Action Powers. Another function is to straighten and color the primitive image formed on the retina. Manas works only in 2D, not 3D. The 3D map is the work of Ahankaara. | |

In the Anthakarana, the intellect is the psychological component that allows knowing what apparently is unknown. The innate ability to identify different objects and the ability to categorize by abstract concepts are some of the functions of the intellect. It is the tool to understand the world.

The ego is the psychological component that differentiates the being from the rest of the universe. This separation is, of course, an illusion. It is a psychological mechanism that brings the ego to entities identified in Prakriti so they recognize themselves as different from everything else.

The mind is the psychological component that can integrate the tools of perception and action. The mind controls the senses, sensation, locomotion, speech, etc. It is also responsible for managing the network of thoughts.

These three elements, we have outlined in a very simplified way here, make up the Antahkarana or inner psychic organ. Antahkarana is a triune organ that essentially integrates limitations of knowledge, will and action. Through this body is made interaction with the world we call "real".

## Antakarana Symbol

As for the symbol that represents it, is composed of three strokes similar to a seven, each representing one of the three aspects, intellect, ego and mind that make the Anthakarana. The figure also recalls a hexahedron or cube, which shows only three of its six sides. Symbolically visible faces represent the three aspects of Buddhi, Ahankaara, Manas while hidden faces represent the divine aspects of Shakti which are the unlimited powers of Knowledge, Will and Action. Thus the Antahkarana symbol energetically establishes a connection between both sides of the Maya veil, freeing up the limitations of this plane with the unlimited power.

This symbol is multidimensional. At first glance appears to be two-dimensional, consisting of three sevens on a flat surface. Each of these seven represents the seven chakras, the seven colors and the seven notes of the musical scale. From another perspective, the symbol looks like a three dimensional cube. Its energy moves from two to three dimensions that can be seen, but also continues through unseen dimensions all the way to the higher vibrations of the Higher.

### Origin

While this is one of the symbols used in ceremonies, rituals and Tibetan systems, it is clear that the Tibetans did not originate the symbol and there are no written records of its true origin.

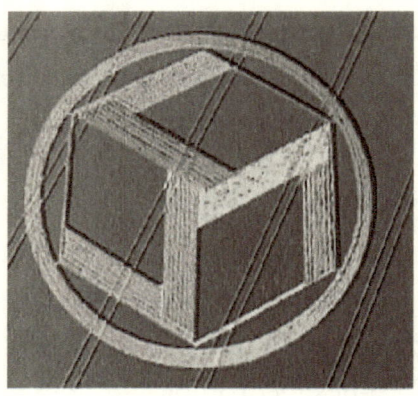

The image above is a photo of the symbol Antahkarana taken in the English countryside. The same corresponds to one of the many crop circles that have been appearing for years mainly in Britain.

These drawings can only be properly appreciated from the air, due to its large size. They usually appear in areas cultivated with cereals such as wheat. The drawings are formed by twisting the stems of plants similar to what happens with velvet, so at a distance can be observed in different color areas.

In its proportions and the speed with which these images appear, usually overnight, it is believed that it is impossible to be made by human beings. Many researchers suggest that these strange drawings are messages sent by light beings from other dimensions or from outer space. As a curious note, it has been observed that crooked stems continue to grow and bear fruit, even said to have a higher yield than the rest.

After this information, the analytical and the mysterious and magical esoteric, I can only leave to its discernment any assessment about the origin and meaning of the symbol Antahkarana. I also recommend you become familiar with the symbol in its practice; that you know and understand how it works and how you can lean on it to enhance and focus your own personal power.

## Types of Antahkarana

For the purpose of its use in the Usui Tibetan Reiki, there are four mandala presentations of the Antahkarana symbol as outlined below:

### Male Antahkarana

The Antahkarana symbol is small. It is used for more direct and powerful healing, as is typical of male energy. It is also useful for meditation, for the mandala of crystals and to remember dreams.

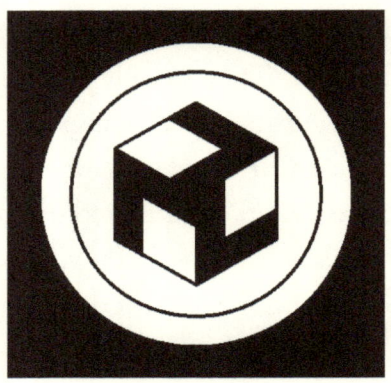

## *Female Antahkarana*

The Antahkarana symbol is big. Healing is softer and more loving. It is very useful for Reiki therapies, since it expands the aura and protects pacient and Reiki practitioner.

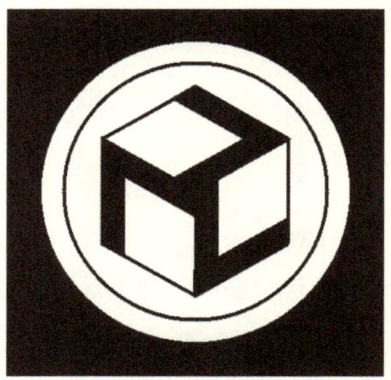

## *Antahkarana Cross*

It purifies and cleans. It helps opening the heart chakra, moving towards unconditional love and compassion. It facilitates the harmonization of the seven chakras.

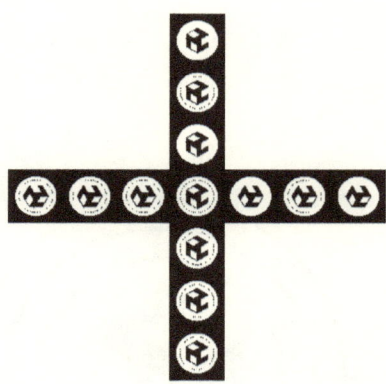

## Multiple Antahkarana

Unlock lower vibrating stuck energies. It is a dispersing symbol in nature. I should not be placed for a long time, only at the beginning of the Reiki treatment, since it can get to disperse energy healing itself.

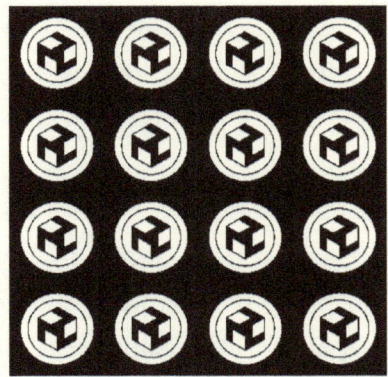

## Sutratma

The Sutratma in its construction is based on the symbol Antahkarana. This mandala generates energy and vitality, promotes longevity and increases physical health while raising the body's defenses. It can be used in conjunction with a mandala Antahkarana in initiations and meditations, one under each foot,

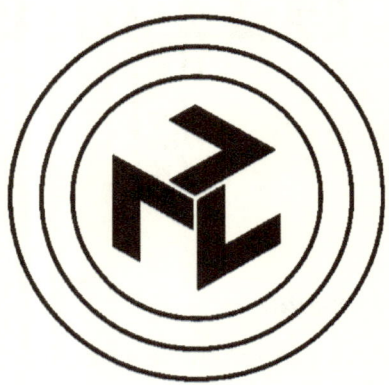

## Uses of the Antahkarana

The Antahkarana mandala is very old and has been widely used for meditation and healing in Tibet and China for thousands of years. It is said to be very powerful. Just by its presence, you can create a positive effect on the chakras and aura.

When doing healing work, this symbol concentrates, focuses and deepens the actions of the energies involved.

When meditating with the mandala on your person or near you, it activates what Taoists call Great Microcosmic Orbit, causing psychic energies, which normally enter the crown chakra, to enter through the feet and travel to the crown by the back of the body and then descend through the front back to the feet. In this way the person is connected with earth, creating a continuous flow of energy through the chakras.

Some recommendations when using Antahkarana are:

- Neutralize the negative energy that has been stuck in objects such as jewelry or crystals. This is done by placing the object between two mandalas or simply placing in above or below a mandala.

- Reinforce any healing work including Reiki, placing the mandalas on the couch during the session.

- Harmonize spaces. Just placing the mandala in a room harmonizes the energy from the environment.

- Improve the connection with dreams, putting the mandala under the pillow to have lucid dreams and to remember them when awaking.

- To reinforce the crystal work using the mandala of crystals.

## An experience with Antahkarana

The forms are energy. That's why all forms constantly emit energy patterns. What follows is an experience recounted by Mimi, a friend, a student and colleague of Peru, which demonstrates the powerful effect Antahkarana mandala when it focuses attention.

*"The energy is intelligent and works for itself," said one day the teacher Dunes, and it was something that stuck with me even without understanding it completely. I went to my country house with my symbols and Antahkarana, to practice and learn to do them. Sitting there I devoted myself to the drawing of symbols. I soon noticed that my ability as a draftsman was not so, but my employee, a countryman, who knew only the wisdom of nature and very good artist, he says from afar with his lampa in*

*hand: "Madam, can I help? "I said" why not? "He sat down and started doing different antahkaranas with great skill, as we talked about those drawings.*

*I told him about the occurrence of these forms in the fields in the UK, but did not explain its use. Deta, the name of the 25 year, listened intently while drawing. The conversation was interrupted by the phrase: "Oh what a weird heat! Right lady?" Drawing the last Antahkarana was finished and he walked away apologizing for a while to cool the excess heat that was in the field of Lima. It took a while to come back and when back he says, "Lady, do you know what happens. It hurt a lot but, strangely, I have expelled a kidney stone, ... that they had to operate to take it out, remember? ... lady it came out alone, it's huge ...And I felt half hurt than when I threw the little stones and it's huge!, Don't you believe me ... want to see it? "When he took the piece of paper where he had it wrapped, I was in speechless amazement. It was bigger than my pinkie fingernail.*

*I looked at him, his eyes staring at me inquisitors and said, "Do you think could have been the drawings madam?" I said yes, and in his native natural simplicity of humble connoisseur of the natural laws of the countryside, he smiled. I said, "be grateful, Deta, for the help was given to you." He did so, in his own way and his way ... I neither asked who he thanked.*

# MANDALA OF CRYSTALS

The Mandala of Crystals is one of the most valuable tools for Reiki practitioners once reached Level III of the Usui Tibetan Reiki system.

It is to have a group of crystals symmetrically around a center. Generally, this arrangement of the crystals is performed on an image to enhance energy Mandala with the intention of said Mandala. In the case of Usui Tibetan Reiki, the Antahkarana image is commonly used.

It is known that crystals have the properties to capture, store and radiate energy. Due to its structure, behave as resonators that can handle energies from subtler levels, including the energy of emotions and thoughts. Some crystals are used for channeling vibrations even angelic and archangelic.

In the Usui Tibetan Reiki the mandala of crystals is usually built with quartz crystal. This crystal has, among others, the following characteristics:

- Contains the purity of the Elohim.
- It is related to the energy of Archangel Gabriel.
- It harmonizes and balances all levels.
- It brings more Universal Life Energy to the body, emotions and mind.
- Gives a sense of clarity and purity.
- Clean the auric field.
- Has positive impact on the chakras.
- It improves mental activity. It amplifies the thoughts.
- Very good tool for deprogramming and reprogramming.
- Detoxifies.
- Clarifies the vision, hearing, thinking and expression.
- Balances the Nervous System.

## Mandala Structure

The mandala of crystals is formed with eight quartz crystals. Seven of them must have a minimum length of 5 inches, elongated shape and ending in a point in one of its ends. Six of these crystals are located in each of the six corners of the hexagon forming Antakarana symbol, with the tips pointing inward. The seventh is called crystal glass master and is located in a corner of the mandala.

The eighth crystal is used to place it in the center of the Mandala and preferably should be in the form of a pyramid.

This last crystal acts as an amplifier and energy resonator that is programmed into the mandala.

The mandala can be on a box where photos and / or various requests are placed. Behind each picture or request Reiki symbols must be placed. As an alternative or complement, the symbols can be placed within the box.

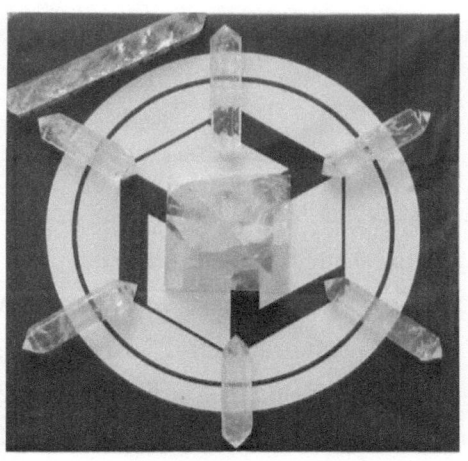

## Selection and preparation of crystals

A very important factor is the choice of the crystals. In addition to following the suggestions listed above, the crystals should be selected personally by at least one of the creators of the mandala. Each crystal has a unique vibrational overtones and affinity between the crystals and the Reiki practitioner must be present in this selection. Follow your intuition when choosing each crystal. As a master crystal you can choose the one with best vibration from the seven crystals. You can even choose a slightly larger crystal for this purpose.

The central crystal is usually of greater volume than others. Although it is not a pyramid, should be a crystal that appeals to you, that you feel or intuit its ability to radiate.

It is important to choose only crystal quartz crystals, being careful not to be confused with smoky quartz. It has been reported that the smoky quartz, although it can channel certain high frequencies, it is also prone to channel low-frequency vibrations that can decrease the power of the mandala.

Once the crystals are chosen proceed to clean with the system of your choice. Following few existing cleaning systems we recommend:

1. Place the crystals in a container that holds water with sea salt. Do this with the intention that the crystals are equipped to receive the purest vibration of love.
2. Expose the container for 24 hours to sunlight and the energy of the moon. If it is Full Moon much better.
3. Remove crystals, washed in running water and preferably dry with a cotton cloth.

## Programming the Mandala

After selecting and cleaning the crystals proceed to place them on the mandala in the position shown in the following figures. Following the programming process consisting of:

- Activate the crystals one by one, holding it between your hands, drawing and applying Reiki symbols for three minutes. After that it is put back into position in the Antahkarana. The master crystal is the last to be activated.
- Take the master crystal in the dominant hand and from the crystal in the center, stroke is made towards the

crystal at the periphery, clockwise from there to the next and from there to the center crystal again as if you were cutting a cake.

- As you make these strokes, visualize the light flowing through the master crystal, connecting all the crystals and letting them radiate light. You can repeat an invocation to attract the energy of love, light and divine wisdom to any process that will assist with the mandala.

- This programming or activation lasts for 72 hours, after which the mandala must be activated again.

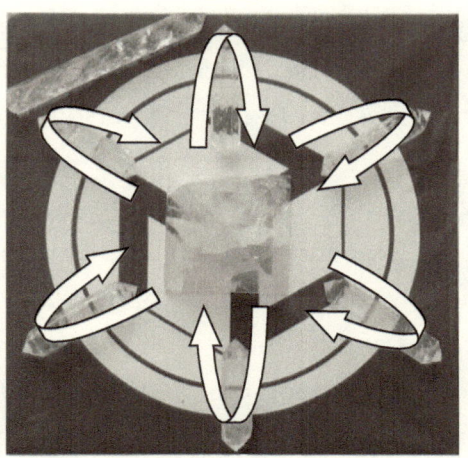

## Uses of the Mandala of Crystals

The energy that is handled in the mandala is very powerful and there is no limit to the number of petitions that can be addressed at once. You can send Reiki to a large number of people simultaneously and permanently. Therefore it is said that in some cases the effect of the mandala is even higher than in the present Reiki.

Nor are there limits on the types of requests that can be placed. The limit is the imagination and creativity of the Reiki practitioner.

It should be clarified that Reiki energy intervenes in processes facilitating its most appropriate solution. In no case should Reiki be taken as a facilitator of personal whims. To better explain this, let us take the case of a person who is dying because of a serious illness. We chose to put this person in the mandala with the intention to help in his process. We can take this action with the expectation that the person heals, but there is other likely scenario and that is the person dies, so abandoning all suffering. Both scenarios are possible and we are not able to decide these issues for the person or change her life choices.

By putting people in the mandala of crystal we are just going to pour energy of love and grace on the situation, so the most appropriate outcome takes place that according to his contract of life, their choices and harmony with the universe and with all parties involved. If the person dies does this mean that Reiki did not work? By no means, it is clear that the result would be the most appropriate, either healing or death. Reiki serves in any case to facilitate the ongoing process.

# MEDITATIONS

The word meditation is used commonly to refer to the function of thinking actively and focused on something or someone. A better word for this type of activity could be reflexion or just thinking.

Another approach to the term meditation, common in esoteric groups and New Age, is to use it as a substitute for visualization term. Visualization is an exercise in which you perform a mental representation of an object, place, situation, person, etc. These visualizations usually are guided by a facilitator or a recording, where a script is narrated aloud to lead the group or the individual to a certain experience.

Meditate is neither thinking nor visualize. The point of meditation is to reach a state of no-mind, which is quite opposite to the reflexion and visualization. It is a state where all thoughts disappear. A state can only be achieved in deep relaxation. Therefore, meditation is the opposite of thinking or reflexion and also separated from visualization.

However, in many cases, given the difficulty for modern man to achieve the state of meditation, visualization is used as a resource or a bridge to meditation. With a proper visualization a relaxed state of mind can be reached, which eventually, will take the person to the meditative state of no-mind.

The visualization can act as a bridge to meditation, when you succeed ignoring it. You only use it as a resource, as an excuse to quiet your mind, just before embarking on the journey to yourself. In fact, meditation itself is just another excuse, another tool. It is a path to achieve awareness of our inner being, is a way to arouse our attention and our consciousness. Once you are aware you do not need meditation. If you are alert, if you are focused, entrenched in yourself, if life is basically beautiful no matter what is happening, if you're happy with yourself, then you do not need meditation. Then you are healed.

The following sections are going to use the word meditation to keep alive the true purpose behind the visualization.

## Anapana Meditation

This is a very old, very simple and very effective method to approach the meditative state.

I.  It begins by taking a comfortable position, you can do it lying down, sitting or standing. As long as you feel comfortable, what you choose is well.

II.  Then a cycle is practiced at least five deep breaths in four phases to increase our capacity to receive the qi from the air.

III.  During these breaths should be observed as the air goes in and out through your nose.

When breathing in, you feel its graze in your nostrils, when breathing out feel its touch in your nostrils. Feel its temperature, its texture, its speed, its intensity.

IV.   Then let the breathing go flowing normally and continue to observe only the air that enters and leaves your nostrils. Do nothing, just watch and let the observer, the presence, appears in you.

V.   If thoughts come up it is fine, just do not give them importance. Do not pay attention! All your attention is focused on breathing in and breathing out through your nose.

## Antahkarana Meditation

Following, we describe the classic meditation with Antahkarana and Reiki symbols who conduct Tibetan lamas:

*The Tibetan meditation practice that uses Antahkarana takes place in a candlelit room. In the middle of the room there is a large oval earthen vessel symbolizing the cosmic egg of the universe. The vessel contains several inches of water and in the middle there is a stool. In the seat of the stool, inlaid in silver, is the symbol of Antahkarana. One wall is covered with copper, polished like a mirror. On the opposite wall there is hanging a tapestry with Reiki symbols.*

*A meditative Tibetan Lama sits on the stool and stares at the image of the Reiki symbols reflected in the copper mirror. This meditation will create a precision in the mind of the one meditating, uniting the consciousness with the transcendental energies of the Reiki symbols, while the symbol on the stool Antahkarana will focus the energies generated to flow evenly through all the chakras and connecting them to earth.*

In our case, can be bits difficult to recreate a scenario like this, however, you can take ideas from this classic meditation and make our own versions. Following some examples:

- Place your feet on the Antahkarana mandala and focus yur gaze on the male DKM symbol, while letting go all thoughts
- Place your feet on the Antahkarana mandala and fix your gaze on the center of another Antakarana mandala, while letting go all thoughts. In this case we may be attracted to the center of the hexahedron, which will increase in size and it can start rotating.
- Perform Anapana meditation with your feet on the Antahkarana mandala.

The most important thing is that everything is made as an accessory to meditation, serve as a resource that facilitates you reach that state of inner peace, a sense of unity that completely heals and frees.

# ENERGY SURGERY

Energy surgery is a procedure that can be done for you or for someone else. The most common is that the Reiki practitioner performs it on other people and looks for a Reiki therapist to perform the surgery on him, should it be needed.

The epistemological basis of this procedure lies in the idea that all diseases that manifest in the physical body have their origin in subtle bodies as the etheric, emotional and mental. Essentially a disease is an imbalance or blockage of energy in one of the subtle bodies that plunges into the physical body.

Many actions and low vibration thoughts with which we resonate daily generate amorphous energy patterns incompatible with human design, invading and blocking the path of chakras and auric bodies. If these patterns are not released properly, if not allowed to flow, they will end up expressing themselves by resonance, at the level of the physical body.

The energy surgery technique is very old and has been practiced in various cultures throughout the centuries. His arrival at Tibetan Reiki is due to a Reiki master William Lee

Rand, who developed it inspired by the Huna ancient science of the Hawaiian Kahuna.

It relies on the use of the Usui Master symbol Dai Ko Myo, as already studied, meaning "Great Being of the Universe shines on me." It can also mean "Great Bright Light", which is a Zen expression to our own true nature of Buddha. Used at the highest level of healing, it exposes the thought that our subtle bodies are a template for our physical body. Thus, when we are sick, the disease is originally formed in our subtle bodies. Dai Ko Myo clean and heal these bodies.

The energy that a Level III Reiki practitioner handles with the use of this symbol, allows healings perform at energy level that may seem amazing to the eyes of the ignorant.

The procedure for performing surgery energy is illustrated below:

## Procedure for Energy Surgery

Firstly must have similar environmental conditions which are used for a Reiki treatment. Also you must have a candle near the massage table, to send to it all that it is detached from the operation with the intention of it being transmuted.

Masculine, feminine and cross Antahkarana mandalas are placed under the massage table. The multiple or mosaic mandala stands apart, on a table, before starting the surgery and once the aura of the patient is bath, it is turned down. We recommend placing the male Antahkarana directly under the area where you intend to intervene.

The steps to be followed during a Reiki surgery are listed below:

I. Perform Ken Yo Ku.

II. Draw in hands masculine DKM, CKR symbols

III. Apply on your own body the CKR symbol, from seventh chakra to the root chakra, as if it would be applied by another person. Also draw CKR in each chakra from 1st to 7th.

IV. Clean the place with CKR symbol; to four walls, floor and ceiling.

V. Place the patient on heart centering and bath the aura.

VI. Place patient's hands to the sides and apply the male DKM symbol on crown chakra, on the front, from the sixth chakra to the root chakra and the soles of his feet.

VII. Ask the patient to expose the reason he had to come for help.

VIII. Ask the patient to locate the physical location of his condition or problem. Can you tell us where it hurts, or any symptoms to guide us?

IX. Ask the patient to focus on the affected area, visualize his problem telling us about the shape of it. Then he will be asked to give us all descriptive information he may have regarding weight, volume, color, consistency, odor, taste, etc. It is not necessary to be exhaustive; the intention is to integrate the patient to the process while mentally he outlines his discomfort.

X. Instruct the patient to extract all low vibration and negativity from his discomfort. That discordant energy will be sent to the Universe to be transmuted. We ask him to focus on the affected part of his body as he described it and visualize it leaving. It is important he keeps that image in his mind during surgery.

XI. Contract Hui Yin and close microcosmic orbit (See Level I).

XII. With hands in front of the face, lengthen the ectoplasm of fingers between 15 and 30 inches. This is done by grasping the fingers one by one and imaginarily stretching them breathing out by mouth emitting an audible sound. These will be the energy scalpels that will be used in surgery. Try to feel them.

XIII. Put your hands before you and draw all the symbols on scalpels with your nose or mentally.

XIV. We proceed to uncover the area of the body to operate and CKR, SHK and DKM male symbols are drawn over the area where the incision will take place.

XV. An incision is made on the skin, it is open and proceed to clean, dig and remove with one hand placing in the other hand what is being removed and blowing it out to the candle with an audible sound.

XVI. If there are well-defined and manageable organs, they are extracted imaginatively and individually cleaned, placing them back in place.

XVII. The temperature of the area is reviewed by placing the palm about 5 inches. If the temperature perceived in the area is very hot or very cold steps XV and XVI should be followed until the temperature is regularized. You can also check the status of the operation with the pendulum.

XVIII. Gather each finger scalpels.

XIX. Draw male DKM, SHK y CKR in the area under surgery.

XX. Close the wound imitating the medical-surgical process and bath the wound with hand without touching the skin.

XXI. Draw again male DKM, SHK y CKR in the area operated.

XXII. Seal chakras, giving a blow in the air with the palm on each one of them.

XXIII. Repeat step VI.

XXIV. Bath the aura again.

XXV. Release Hui Yin and open microcosmic orbit (See Level I).

XXVI. Separate from the patient.

XXVII. Perform Ken Yo Ku, this time giving thanks for the process to masters and beings of light who assisted you.

Steps XV y XVI require full attention from Reiki practitioner, since he must visualize or imagine as clearly as possible what he is doing. After this process the practitioner must clean hands, either by washing, strongly shaking them or passing them through the heat of the fire, as it is done in the Reiki treatments.

The patient should stay on the stretcher few minutes to recover from surgery. Also be advised not to bath in the next 12 hours. He is also notified that he may experience a healing crisis as feeling discomfort in the operated area, have diarrhea, dizziness or overall malaise. In reality, all these symptoms are indicative of body's favorable reaction to the intervention.

When surgery is complete, a full session of Reiki is done suggesting the patient to get four to six additional treatments, preferably on consecutive days for a better result of the operation.

In cases with chronic conditions It is recommended applying Reiki during 21 consecutive days after the operation; some present treatments can be combined with remote treatments.

Interventions may be repeated depending on the result obtained.

# RE-POLARIZATION

## Wounds and Meridians

One of the most healing method used by modern medicine is the surgical intervention. However it is important to note that surgery is studied in medicine as traumatism, given its invasive nature and imbalances that inevitably occur during surgery. When studying the changes that this technique can cause to health and the balance of the human body, allows to be used as a healing method with a level of controlled traumatism.

Some physical body changes caused by surgery and other traumatic injuries are: loss of body cell mass, edema, acid-base imbalance, cardiac involvement, risk of infection, impaired renal function, among other. Most of these possible effects are controlled and monitored during surgery and in the postoperative period, evolving very well in most cases without additional complications.

Just as surgery creates imbalances in the physical body, also creates imbalances in the subtle bodies. This is especially evident in the etheric body which produces measurable changes in the energy circuits known as meridians. When evaluating with Dermatron the energy resonators on both sides of a scar, whether it is surgical or not, it is easy to detect altered values in the acupuncture meridians crossing said scar. If this energy dysfunction situation last longer, it will end up interfering the flow of local and / or distal energy in the areas and tissues furnished with the affected meridians.

## The solution

One way to prevent this energy imbalance is perpetuated in time is to perform a procedure known as re-polarization of the wound. There are several methods devised by alternative medicines to achieve re-polarization and restoring the normal flow in the meridians, among which we can mention:

Neural Re-polarization

Electric Re-polarization

Re-polarization by Gems

In addition to these methods, this book includes a method of re-polarization using Reiki energy and crystals.

### *Method of Reiki Re-polarization*

The method consists of four Reiki treatments that can be performed at intervals not exceeding one week and not less than one day between sessions. It is recommended that this procedure is performed three months after surgery. The steps are as follows:.

I.     Placing several crystals along the wound with a gap of about 1 centimeter or more, depending on the size of each crystal. The crystals should be black tourmaline. In the absence of the former quartz crystal is used.

II.   Immediately, carry out all the steps to start a Reiki treatment.

III.   Just before starting with positions draw the male DKM on the scar.

IV.   Apply one or more positions on the scar, depending upon size thereof, during 6 minutes each. No need to touch the patient. With hands two or three inches from the skin will be working in the etheric body while radiating crystals to amplify Reiki energy.

V.   Again apply male DKM over the scar.

VI.   Complete the treatment as it is done with any conventional Reiki treatment.

VII.  After hands are withdrew, the patient stays six more minutes with crystals on the scar.

VIII. Remove the crystals.


Note that no conventional positions of Reiki are performed. It's just the scar, although the whole process of opening and closing of the session is fully respected.

# RETURN TO HOME

At the time of disincarnating, Reiki gives us the opportunity to help the one leaving, so that with a more harmonious transit. This is an activity commonly performed by a worker of dreams. Dreams workers accompany people in their departure, helping them to prepare the way before leaving the physical plane and staying with them during and after physical death.

Moribund

The person, who is near death, can receive great benefits from Reiki. On the physical level it can help to alleviate or endure pain and hardship to which the person may be subject.

In the emotional and mental plane Reiki can be of great value. In many cases death scares, as everything is unknown. Peace and transcendental extra-physical contact is perceived during a Reiki treatment, can be useful to help calm fears and anxiety. It can also facilitate internal connections and / or spiritual to facilitate acceptance of the transition process.

In these cases it is recommended to apply daily present and / or distant Reiki treatments, taking into account the following specific recommendations:

- Use female, male and cross Antahkarana mandalas.
- Draw every symbol on the patient: CKR, SHK, HSZSN and male DKM before going hands on and after sealing the chakras.
- Do an extra position on the crown chakra. In this case, the male DKM is applied apart in this chakra and visualizing how it penetrates accompanied by an intense violet light. One of the positions of the head can be replaced by this.
- During the treatment, visualize the person involved in light and determined and happy walking into the light. Combine shades of gold, silver and violet for this visualization.

## After Death

This is a moment of special importance for the soul. Depending on the life experiences, beliefs, fears, characteristics of death and many other conditions, discarnate souls may find it difficult to follow their way back Home.

It is appropriate that at close moments after death a special Reiki treatment is performed to support the soul's journey into light. This is a beautiful work that was done in other ages with great dedication and lots of love, joy and much celebration, by the workers of dreams.

This session features short Distant Reiki with respect to its ritual (see Level II). However, the difference lies in the intense visualization and blessings sent to the departed soul, the honor that she receives and the support that is given during her return.

For this special Distant Reiki treatment the following ideas are suggested:

- Use male DKM.
- Work with the soul of the person with hands on the male Antahkarana.
- When sending Reiki, visualize the soul of the person walking a beautiful lit path, beautifully decorated, as you would imagine it would be for you or you think the person would like.
- Accompany the person through that path. Encourage her, joke with her, give her confidence. Talk to her about her impeccability and her magnificence.
- Tell her that on the other end of the path there are angels waiting, and not to be afraid of the light.
- At some point you will have to let him go and observe as this trusting soul advances towards the light, to the angelic family meeting.

On successive days this type of special sessions can be repeated following intuition of Reiki practitioner. You can also make several Distant Reiki treatments in celebration of the soul, with a clear message in mind: Do not fear the Light.

# BEYOND REIKI

As of my relationship with Reiki and after initial adjustments at all levels, a whole new universe opened for me. In essence I felt a cool breeze, as eye drops, which has cleared up my look, my vision of things.

As a result of this renewed clarity of perception, different concepts and systems for energy handling, have arisen, or I may say emerge from intuition, with the intention to be disseminated and practiced by those who so wish.

Some of these systems that I have been able to shape are listed below, first, as a way to make clear of what can be achieved with Reiki in the development of intuition; second, to introduce the reader to these methods, which will be the subject of future developments.

## GeoReiki

GeoReiki is a healing system that works from non-polarity. It aims to restore balance in our bodies without acting in favor or against any of the poles.

It is common, to find therapies whose line of treatment is to weaken some energy pattern identified as undesirable or to boost some kind of energy that it is weakened. These two modes of action fit perfectly with conventional medicine, as well as alternative therapies. When prescribing antibiotics, allergenic, surgery or radiation, in allopathy; when discussing about sedating the kidney or toning the liver in acupuncture; when infusion of cayenne is recommended to counteract insomnia; in all these cases, we are applying an action in just one direction, based on our judgment about what needs to be enhanced or suppressed.

Systems that work like this are highly elaborated and require a lot of information and knowledge to make responsible decisions, because for every action there is always a reaction. Yet the result is not guaranteed 100%, because the variables involved are endless and cannot be taken into account, all at once.

GeoReiki is an alignment system that combines Reiki channeling with clay to potentiate the effect of balancing and facilitate healing. One of the main benefits of this system is that both clay and Reiki are smart energies and are not polarized. This allows them to be used interchangeably to sedate or tone, to soothe or stimulate.

In any case, the practitioner makes decisions choosing the direction of polarity in which to work.

The training includes simple and effective teaching techniques of exploration that facilitate application of this therapy.

## Tattva Healing

Tattva Healing is a system of healing that invites harmonize our bodies according to the higher states of Being.

This is accomplished by connecting from the physical and etheric with sensory patterns like shape, sound and color. These patterns operate as harmonics of the higher levels of Being, fostering resonance and harmonization required by all bodies and chakras.

Tattva Healing integrates hands-on, mudras and mantras, sacred forms, chambers of healing and vital ethers, among other resources, to adjust the energy balance and strengthen the connection to the higher planes of our being. Tattwa Healing can impact markedly increased levels of consciousness.

## Life Mastery

You were taught Math, Spanish, Chemistry and more, but no one taught you what about this phenomenon called life. Now is a good time to take some notes about that pending subject.

The focus of this training is to stimulate a shift in perception that may lead to a change in the level of consciousness. Keys and tools are given so you can use to effectively support your personal evolution process. In this case Reiki is an invaluable tool, because it is a faithful companion when reprogramming your mind and body with the new patterns we want to incorporate.

We propose a radical change of paradigms about reality, in which the duality begins to give way to the triality, as a central view of all the processes and phenomena of the universe.

# ADDENDA

# HUMAN ENERGY STRUCTURE

The human body is a complex energy organization, whose most obvious manifestation to the senses is the physical body. But there is a statement that says "things are seldom what they seem" and this saying is very true in the case of Man.

Take the case of a television. It is a device with a certain physical structure that works only when power is supplied and if the contrary happens the TV operation will stop. Similarly, the physical body of man requires energy to function properly. When the energy flow is stopped in our body we simply die and the physical body becomes a corpse. Unlike the TV, the human body is composed of organic matter, making it highly attractive to millions of living organisms. In the absence of the high vibration energy barrier that protects the physical body, these millions of beings take over the food that an inert body provides for them.

Where were all those millions of microorganisms capable of decomposing a body in few months? They were in the environment looking for suitable habitat to feed on and proliferate. The living human body is not suitable for them because of its high frequency energy; instead, a corpse, is a paradise for these beings.

The human body is an energy structure system where they interlock to form a cohesive unit. These structures are known for millennia and have been studied both in East and West. In short we can say that this energy system consists of three basic components:

- The chakras or energy centers. These are vortices rotating of energy arranged in different points of the human anatomy.

- The subtle bodies (aura). They are energy bodies accompanying the physical body, containing it, wrapping it and interpenetrating it. These bodies are collectively known as the aura. Its existence has been proven experimentally with psychics, as well as with special equipment such as camera Kirlian or GDV.

- The nadis or energy channels. They form a network of intangibles "arteries and capillaries". Its role is to lead vital energy through non-material energy system. A well-known subset of this system of canals, which operates at the etheric level, is the acupuncture meridians.

The three elements are perfectly interconnected. The chakras connect the nadis receiving and sending energy through them. Networks of Nadis penetrate subtle bodies, while the chakras are expressed in each of the bodies, serving as connecting element and coordinator.

## Chakras

The chakras are located where energy lines cross the nadis. There are different types of chakras and their importance varies depending on the amount of energy line crossings (see Table Chakras Classification on the next page).

The chakras receive and store primary energy through the vortex and distribute it to the nadis and meridians, from there to the nervous system and the endocrine system, then the blood, cells and all body atoms.

Each chakra has four main functions:

- energize the auric layers
- feed the psychological function
- feed the physiological function
- transmit the energy among auric layers

## Clasification of Chakras

| Group of Chakras | Description |
| --- | --- |
| Chakra of Supra-Consciousness | Appears above the crown chakra. In this chakra the energy lines are crossed 49 times. |
| 7 Major Chakras | They are located along the spinal column. Appear where they cross 28 times the energy lines. |
| 3 Chakras of Physical-Psychic Vitality | These chakras are the splenic, located at the height of the spleen, another located at the height of the stomach and a third at the height of the 7th cervical. Appear where the energy lines are crossed 21 times. |
| 18 Minor Chakras | These Chakras are located in the following areas of the body: Eyes (2), Ears (2); Sternum; Chest (2); Diaphragm; Pancreas; Liver; Groin (2); Hands (2), Knees (2); Feet (2). Appear where the energy lines are crossed 14 times. |
| 60 Chakras of Physical Balance | They are bilateral, so they really are 120. Here the energy lines are intersected 7 times. These points correspond to the Old Su points of the Traditional Chinese Medicine. |

## *Cords*

The cords can be defined as energy lines or threads that connect the chakras of two individuals. This connection usually represents a warning or a cry for help from one person to the other. This is an unbalanced exchange energy, where one person thrives, feeds or supports another. This can lead to severe damage to both parties, because it inhibits the development of the chakras on the receiver and drains the life energy in the giver.

The cords have a specific meaning for each chakra. That meaning helps to describe the nature of the relationships we establish with others. Similarly, to identify the relationships we have with others, we know what kind of cords we are establishing with them and which can be affected chakras.

The connection to the outside using chakras should be through heart chakra exclusively. This limits the possibility of generating dependency or any other type of unbalanced situations. Communication through the heart chakra expresses unconditional love we feel towards all creation and is the most balanced connection that we have with others and with our environment.

Following is a brief explanation of the higher chakras characteristics.

## Major Chakras

The major chakras are the most known and studied since they are the most important for human energy balance. In this section we will refer exclusively to these major chakras.

Vortices of major chakras connect the central nadi called sushumna, which is located vertically between the base and crown chakras. Each chakra is actually a group of concentric chakras, expressed in each auric body. So when we speak of a chakra, we are actually talking about seven concentric chakras, one for each body.

Physiologically, each chakra is related to an endocrine gland. On the psychological level, it appears that the development of a chakra is associated with different emotions. Anatomically relationships between organs and body parts and chakras are observed. In turn, each chakra relates to a group of pathologies that can be treated balancing the chakra.

## *First Chakra: Basic*

Location: At the apex of the sacrum, between the anus and sexual organs.

Sanscrit Name: MULADHARA

Grand: Suprarenal

Emotion: Rage

Color: Red

Musical Note: DO

Sound: LAM

Cords: I want you to help me survive. It expresses a dependency on the basics, food, basic needs of shelter and protection.

It is linked with earthly existence, with survival. It has to do with physical energy and desires to live. It has to do with the ability to get food, economic resources, employment, desires, independence of others, etc.

## Second Chakra: Umbilical

Location: Sacral region below the navel.
Sanskrit Name: SVADHISHTHANA
Gland: Gonad
Emotion: Lust
Color: Orange
Musical Note: RE (D)
Sound: VAM
Cords: I am interested in you sexually. Give me your emotional support, pay attention to my emotions.

It is linked to the reproduction, propagation of the species and sexual pleasure. It is useful in treating diseases of Reproductive System. It is also related to other characteristics such as curiosity, creative searching of material pleasure, and a taste for art, beauty, emotions and relationships with others.

## Third Chakra: Solar Plexus

Location: Below the lower level of the shoulder blades; in the area of the diaphragm, above the stomach (in the pit of the stomach).
Sanskrit Name: MANIPURA
Gland: Pancreas
Emotion: Arrogance
Color: Yellow
Musical Note: MI (E)
Sound: RAM
Cords: I want some of your energy, not just mine. I rather operate with your energy than to be responsible for my own. I want to control you.

Represents the personality, the Ego, the will to know and learn. It has to do with communicating with the desire to live. It is the point of connection with others and is also of great importance in self-acceptance.

## Fourth Chakra: Heart

Location: Between the shoulder blades. It is in the area of the heart.

Sanskrit Name: ANAHATA
Gland: Thymus
Emotion: Selfishness, Hatred
Color: Green
Musical Note: FA
Sound: YAM
Cords: I love you, I like you.

Unconditional love, capacity of love freely and without conditions.

## Fifth Chakra: Throat

Location: Behind the neck, in the nape, reaching upward to the medulla oblongata; In the middle of the throat in the Adam's apple.

Sanskrit Name: VISHUDDHA
Gland: Thyroid and parathyroid
Emotion: Addiction
Color: Light Blue
Musical Note: SOL
Sound: HAM

Cords: I want to communicate with you. I want to talk to you.

It involves communication, creativity, sound, ability to receive and assimilate, palate, hearing and smell.

## Sixth Chakra: Frown

Location: In the cavity formed by the Turkish saddle of the sphenoid bone. It is in the eyebrows, just above the eyes and in the midline of the forehead.
Sanskrit Name: AJNA
Gland: Pituitary
Emotion: Envy
Color: Indigo Blue
Musical Note: LA
Sound: OM
Cords: You have someone in your head, thinking hard on yourself or wondering what you're thinking, or what you think of him or her.

It is related to intuition, clairvoyance and the hearing, in the field of the paranormal.

## Seventh Chakra: Crown

Location: At the top of the head.
Sanskrit Name: SAHASRARA
Gland: Pineal
Emotion: All emotions
Color: White, Golden, Violet
Musical Note: SI
Sound: -

Cords: I want to control you. I want you to follow my teachings.

It is the link between the spiritual mind and the physical brain. It is the connection to the higher spirituality of the human being.

## Aura

The set of energy bodies coexisting with the physical body in the same space and surround is called Aura. Generally there are seven high vibrational energy bodies covering and coexisting with the physical body:

- The ethereal body.
- The emotional body.
- The mental body.
- The astral body.
- The body of the ethereal pattern
- The celestial body
- The causal body.

Each of these bodies has its own energy frequency band. The ethereal body, which is the closest to the physical body, vibrates with the lowest frequency range. The upper bodies have increasing frequency bands.

### *The Ethereal Body*

The ethereal body has roughly the same size and shape as the physical body. Thus it is also called ethereal double. It contains the vital energy of the organs, tissues, glands and meridians of acupuncture. This body vitalizes and sustains the physical body until death. It is formed in each reincarnation and dissolves at three to five days of physical death.

This body receives energy through the chakras of the solar plexus and spleen. It accumulates these energies and it continuously leads them to the physical body to balance cellular level. The energy stored in this body is radiated out through the chakras and pores, forming a protective aura around the physical body, which prevents pathogens and contaminants penetrate the physical body.

Hence it is said that a person cannot get sick because of external causes. The reason for an illness lies always in itself. The thoughts, emotions and a way of life that is not in line with the body's natural needs (overwork, unhealthy food, alcohol, nicotine and drugs), can weaken and consume vital ethereal energy.

Before manifesting in the physical body, diseases manifest themselves in the ethereal body, which can be detected and treated at this level.

Ethereal and physical bodies react very well to the pulses coming from the mental body. This could be the successes in health using mental techniques. A great impact on health can be achieved with suitable suggestions.

The etheric also acts as an intermediary between the higher energy bodies and physical body. It transmits to the emotional body and the mental body information that is collected through the bodily senses and simultaneously transmits energy and information from the higher bodies to the physical body.

One of the most interesting and most studied parts of the etheric is the system of meridians of Traditional Chinese

Medicine, one of the cornerstones in the study of the human energy anatomy.

## Emotional Body

The emotional body, often also called astral body is the carrier of our feelings, our emotions and qualities of our character. Every emotion will radiate through the emotional body. For example, emotions like anxiety, anger, oppression and worry generate in the aura dark nebulae figures. The more a person opens his consciousness to love, surrender and joy, clearer and transparent colors are emotional aura radiating.

Feelings not released from the emotional body tend to perpetuate and grow. In this way a person usually repeats, again and again, situations that attract emotional vibrations of unreleased feelings. The frequency of anger in a person attracts situations where his anger is confirmed over and over.

Emotional structures continue to exist through the various incarnations if not released, since the emotional body survives after physical death and joins in reincarnation with new physical and ethereal bodies. The unreleased experiences stored in the emotional body partly determine the circumstances of the new life.

## Mental Body

The thoughts and ideas and rational and intuitive knowledge are in the mental body. Its vibration is greater than the ethereal body and the emotional body.

The more alive the thoughts are and the more profound the intellectual knowledge of a person is, the clearer and intense are the colors that radiate your mental vehicle.

At its lowest frequency, this body has to do with rational thought. These thoughts are mostly related to aspects of the material world, personal wellness and rational approach to problem solving.

In its highest frequency, the mental body is a true integrator that receives and interprets the universal truths and integrates with rational understanding. This allows humans to be aware of the true nature of things.

## *The Higher Bodies*

So far the description of related bodies Human physical appearance. The ethereal, emotional and mental bodies are expressed and manifest physically. The astral body is the link between the physical and spiritual aspects of man. The higher bodies, including the astral, do not get sick. That's why during the healing practice greater attention is paid to work with the lower bodies related to the physical world.

# QUESTIONS AND ANSWERS

In this chapter some of my answers and comments on issues of Reiki are expressed. This information is taken from the Light Seekers Forum (http://buscadluz.superforos.com), where I invite you to participate to learn about different disciplines holistic and spiritual development. I thank the friends of the forum, since with their valuable questions have made me dig deeper into various topics of Reiki and healing in general.

The questions and answers have been simplified and adapted to adhere to the topics of Reiki that are relevant for the purposes of this book. The names or other identification of individuals have been suppressed.

## Requirements for Reiki

*I'm with the idea of doing Reiki on my vacation. Now the question is: I need some prior preparation, some special virtue in me. I'm very animated and even excited by just projecting myself and think I'm going to attend the course. I've been a vegetarian for 9 years; does that in some way facilitate the process? I am a neophyte in the matter, for now I'm just starting to read on the subject, what do you think about it?*

Well, there is an emotion that, when present, makes the process smoother, deeper and more complete. That emotion is enthusiasm. Enthusiasm is one of the best ways to approach God, that is, oneself.

Reiki is a great friend who accompanies you to approach the process yourself. The enthusiasm you put does the rest when channeled and becomes intent and responsibility.

You do not require special preparation and if you have a vegetarian diet help, especially since they will experience some symptoms of the cleansing process typically seen in other cases.

I recommend you keep your enthusiasm, but do not hold any expectations. That way you can be more receptive to the process and actually receive what initiation may give you.

Something else I recommend is to not read a lot of Reiki before you are attuned. I know you can be a little anxious and that leads you to anticipate, but that could condition yourself not allowing you to fully receive the message from your teacher.

Have a happy attunement!

*Do you think it would be more advisable to do the 3 levels approximately in month and a half? I think that as you work removing the energies, perhaps do everything at once could be counterproductive. What do you think?*

I recommend you wait between levels. If you have one and half months, I suggest you only follow I and II levels. That can do wonders. In fact that is all that is needed to make regular Reiki sessions traditionally.

Level III of Usui Tibetan introduces energy surgery which is a procedure inherited from the Indians Kahuna of Hawaii. For that kind of work is better have practiced Reiki for a reasonable time, which in most cases is not less than 2 months.

I have seen cases where they have taken Level I and II on consecutive days and then discontinued practicing Reiki because they have found it overwhelming. They have not had time to assimilate and incorporate energetically the whole process.

There has also been the case of students who have complained starting the first level, because they preferred to have done the second immediately instead of waiting the 21 days, etc. However, a week after the attunement, they recognize that it is better that way, because they feel that there are many movements of energy that must be assimilated before proceeding.

Anyway, seek guidance to teachers with whom you want to work and decide what you think is right for you.

## Self-taught Reiki

*I have a fundamental doubt with respect to Reiki. I've seen a lot of information which shows the positions, mandalas and symbols used in Reiki. My question is: If, in short, what a Reiki practitioner does is channeling Reiki universal energy that is everywhere and it's all, is it necessary to learn Reiki from a teacher or facilitator? If a person wants to do Reiki, self-taught, is that possible?*

Yes it is possible. Everything is possible. The issue is how long it would take and how many turns you give to reach a point where you really channel universal energy and do not empathize with the patient energy, i.e. not reflecting imbalances one another.

New generations of children are being born; who probably do not need to pass the initiation process. However, for those of us from previous generations, we are deeply pained walking the path without assistance.

Actually Reiki's attunement path is just initiations for the Reiki practitioner to be purified and healed himself. Imagine we are exquisite bamboo flutes that have been thrown into a quagmire. Before we can issue a consistent note, we must be cleaned. This is the effect of Reiki attunements. They clean our subtle bodies of many blocks, beliefs and limitations for the loving vibration of the universe can be heard through us.

The easiest and harmonious way I know to do that cleansing is through Reiki. That's why Reiki is a gift that comes to support accelerated global growth.

If a person manages to uncover, cleaned through her own means and also manages to make this connection with the universal energy, then for me it is as valid as the Reiki practitioner who has been initiated. After all Dr. Mikao Usui did not initiate another person.

*I fully agree that the Reiki practitioner must study and be initiated, but I am in full disagreement with how expensive these studies have become. For me in particular I wanted to do the master's level, but the costs are in dollars and are over one thousand. In this case, my choices will the Reiki practitioner himself must be attuned but Reiki masters must cut costs down to make it more accessible to interested persons.*

There is something I find curious. You say that "... Reiki masters must cut costs to make it more accessible to interested persons."

The question I ask is how interested are those people? How interested in Reiki? How interested in the money?

Reiki teachers I know, have been interested enough to pay what it costs their Mastery. Lowering costs is to make suitable expertise for those who are so keen NOT to pay all costs.

Part of Mastery may well be a re-evaluation of the relative importance of the spiritual interests and service compared to the importance given to money, don't you think so? What weighs more? What is more important, and what is closer to your passion?

On the other hand, the main purpose for Reiki mastery is initiating others, something that may well constitute a significant part of the income of a Reiki master. If you have a commitment to Reiki teaching, students will come in the most unexpected way and probably investment will be recovered.

So, as personal learning and as a business, the costs of the masteries make much sense, at least from my perspective.

## The Principles of Reiki

*This resonance point you explained to me has helped me a lot. Actually, for some reason, the simple fact of not replying with the same vibrational frequency received from other people or that arises in oneself, is the master key. In practice it may be difficult, but I think the issue is to be aware and try it, right?*

As all, understand this mechanism and apply it, can become the master key to radically change your relationships in life that are not anything but the relationship with yourself. You're already living your own mastery in these things, right?

A fundamental conflict to overcome in these cases is the ego frenzy. As you say, we must be vigilant. If we do not time notice the energy of anger, we begin to resonate and when we realize it has already taken hold of us. At this point, our ego is the master of the situation and is very little we can do. The ideas of humiliation, wounded pride, "self-respect," are enthrone hopelessly in our bodies thus becoming puppets handled by the instincts and low passions...

It's nice that you're doing well with this process ... really nice you are managing your life from a more conscious perspective.

*"The ideas of humiliation, wounded pride, "self-respect," are enthrone hopelessly in our bodies thus becoming puppets handled by the instincts and low passions..." How much material to "shred" contained in this fragment, right?*

Look, I think we've all felt those emotions and we have felt compelled to defend less. We have defended ourselves a thousand ways, each more aggressive than the other. But the result of these confrontations is very poor. One is shaky and very uncomfortable. Other times you feel ashamed for all the way you behaved and wants the earth to swallow you.

Sure we've been trained to react to anything that we think is attacking us, instead of teaching that there is no aggression but self-harm.

Humiliation is something that is felt in front of the actions and opinions of others, but it is one who chooses to feel that. Since somehow we have beliefs that make us vulnerable to such actions or opinions. This has much to do with that we define from what they say about us and how we are treated. It is part of the habit of looking outside us.

The "self-respect" is rather a synonym for pride. Love does not belong to anyone; it's just love and has nothing to do with defense, penalties, barriers or property. We mistreat both the word love that sometimes sounds ridiculous and cheesy in contexts that should serve as inspiration.

Well, our personality, our ego, has been conditioned by the eye for an eye, but we are big enough, right? Nor is it to sit and blame those who came before us by the teachings that were given to us. We know that everyone always does the best he can. Now we have the opportunity to reverse that process for us and as a result, for those who come after. This is part of the magic act that we workers and seekers of the light have to make.

We have tools and we are not alone. The right moment to make a difference is NOW. Do not leave for another Monday, as is usual with these diets you will ever meet.

## Authorization to do Reiki

*I usually use a pendulum along with the practice of Reiki and the first thing I do before giving Reiki or for example, use the pendulum for chakra leveling, is asking for permission. Turns out there is a person (my husband) in particular that when he sometimes is not feeling well and I ask "permission", the same is denied. Have any of you had a case in which permission have been denied to give power to someone? What do you think that could mean?*

I can say that Reiki should not be done without the consent of the person who will receive it. This is a principle that is universal, since it applies not only to Reiki, but to Tarot readings, ERT and many other therapies.

Sometimes it is to go seeking permission to the Higher Self of the person, using the pendulum, tarot, runes, etc. But if it is the case of a person close to you, you can consult them directly.

I'm not sure your situation, or if he has told you he wants Reiki or not, that's why I'm talking in general as I see it.

If you're the one you want to send Reiki and he does not authorize it, you can be treading the slippery slope of disrespecting his free-will.

If he wants, I do not need to use another tool to obtain authorization.

*Do you really feel that the issue "permission" is as "unmovable?" I always feel the good vibes, and beautiful wishes issuing not need permission to send. If such a thing, is not accepted, or not applicable, the other guy has the same power to block ... as we have to send.... do not forget that we talk about energy, not physical third-dimensional manifestation.*

As to what you mention, I think actually there is nothing set in stone. If you want you can send Reiki to people whenever you want. The permit is a recommendation that you can take or leave, because after all it's your free will.

I think you know the genesis of the permit as Reiki rule, but basically, according to legend it was a Usui's personal experience when treating people without that request; what brought him more of a an ungrateful claim by those healed.

This permit has several edges to reflect:

- It is a matter of respect to the free choice of others,
- It's a matter of not throwing pearls before swine,
- It is an issue of personal responsibility of the recipient and sender energy.
- Others

At another level of things, the idea of helping someone with Reiki or any other means, regardless of the will of the person, reminds me this story I summarize below:

"This was a compassionate and kind man that seeing as the butterfly struggled to get out of its cocoon, he armed himself with beautiful wishes and decided to open it himself and thus release the butterfly from such torture. The result of this effort was as expected, the butterfly did not have to do more to get out of its tight dwelling ... However, for the rest of its short life, the butterfly went crawling on the floor, it never managed to develop the necessary strength in its wings to be able to expand them and fly..."

In life, it may be very appropriate to learn not to get carried away by clichés as "good", "ethical", "fair", etc. We can try to be more humble and give space for life to flow and allow each person to choose the way it wants to move, as there is no such thing as "a good way for everyone ".

I hear some Christian text that says something like "The path that leads to hell is paved with good intentions." I do not know, but if we go by the fate of our butterfly...

*I agree with your explanation, thinking about the third dimension, but I have some questions: First, the Reiki to me is not just something that is done on a stretcher, following the usual manual. Second, if I ask permission to lay hands on someone and give him the best "energy possible," then do I understand that I must ask permission to "my enemy" to wish for him light, or send him love? That is, the way I see it is that I do not interfere in the "will" of another subject, I just put at his disposition a tool in which I have faith, and I think he probably needs it and does not know how to ask for it.*

As I said at the beginning of the previous answer, you can do as you like, it is a matter of free will. It seems trivial perhaps, but it is the only thing I can tell you honestly, because that is the only rule of the game of life. Everything else is agreements, conventions, preferences, myths, fears, belief systems and much more, we humans have been creating as we develop the game.

Of course it's due to the use given to our free will that we have gotten where we are, with all the "pros and cons" included. With the use we have done of our free will we have generated karma and dharma, we have built and destroyed and all this has been done in perfect divine order. How is this possible? Well, because the universal energy is self-leveling and compensates with a motion to the right and another to the left. There is no single action and every choice we make changes automatically the state of things in the universe.

Reiki is neither good nor bad, so if you want to send good things you can try something else. The same happens if you want to send bad things. Reiki is self-balanced universal energy and thus self-balancing. Under the influence of Reiki you can expect a marriage to end quickly or miraculously fix, but you cannot guarantee either outcome. The result is given as appropriate. The concepts of good and evil are only human and ethical notions are meaningless in the real balance of things. Reiki has nothing to do with the stories of Indians and cowboys, princesses and witches and princes and villains.

I choose to do Reiki essentially when asked. You can choose to do it when you feel it or you think necessary.

I choose to learn to accept myself by accepting others and I know the rest is done in addition. Thus I avoid identifying other humans as enemies. I have the certainty that we all have all the love of the Source at our disposal. That's why I take care to find it for me, without judging ... I can thereby raise real motivation in others to look for it for themselves through the paths they choose and when they are ready.

Now, while free will is something we established at multidimensional level as a game premise, Reiki is a matter of 4th dimension, as in other dimensions this type of procedure is not relevant. Reiki is a loving way of placing harmonic references so human costumes are balanced with a frequency remembering home. So while the connection is divine, the Reiki experience is only relevant to our 4th dimension.

So I think we can all be happy exercising our free will and taking responsibility for every one of our creations. This is the Age of Responsibility, which invites us to be conscious co-creators with Spirit. Beyond "good and bad", it comes to choosing between being conscious or not. That is what makes the difference between being responsible or not. The good human of the butterfly, is actually a dangerous kind, because behind his craving for goodness covers countless irresponsible and thoughtless behaviors, motivated only by his desire to "do something good".

That being said, I repeat what said before, it is just a matter of free will and any choice you make is perfect in divine order. NO trials. The ups and downs for the humans involved will be lower if you choose consciously and responsibly, but in any case your choice is ALWAYS flawless in the eyes of the Spirit.

## The sensitivity of Reiki

*I am a Level II Reiki practitioner. From the beginning I've noticed that I can perceive the pain or discomfort of the people I deal with. In other occasions I do not need to give them energy, it just happens being in a small place and energies are mixed, allows me to feel what they feel.*

I see you've been very moved by your energy. This can happen because you are very exposed. When the aura is too expanded and responsiveness is very high, empathy or resonance is larger and can have significant consequences.

Draw the symbols to yourself every day to protect your auric field and when doing self-Reiki, use affirmations for your bodies to learn to handle the lower vibrations that you receive, as information and not as resonance.

Some statements that you can use are:

- I am the light
- I choose to resonate with high vibrations
- My bodies are aligned and unified
- My chakras are in perfect harmony

Then you can identify more specific things and incorporate appropriate affirmations to each case.

One more thing. When you listen to another person, hold the center in you. Do not get sucked by the story; do not lose yourself in the story, because that is a way to create empathy. In this case it is happening automatically and you are not doing it consciously, that is why emotions surprise you. You must keep your center, be always an observer.

To better see the difference, I make a parallel with the way of watching a movie. A common spectator dreams and lives the film down to the smallest detail; to the point that when it ends, he has to take time to rearrange his emotions and his thoughts.

A filmmaker sees the movie from another view, attentive to the way that embodies the theme, the characters, the script, special effects, etc. He is aware all the time, not lost in history, not unbalanced. However he very well understands everything that is happening and has a very deep insight of the situation, being able to suggest solutions and consciously learn from the narrative.

Keep going because you have a great gift, just try to be the one using it and not that is disorderly present in your life. You learned to walk dominating your muscles, right? Now learn to use your vision through your attention.

## Reiki and the crisis of Faith

There are few people who have been initiated into Reiki and after a time of more or less successful tests, decide to abandon. This decision is often unconscious, as so many other decisions we make in life. However, the fact that it is unconscious does not mean it is not our responsibility. Being unconscious IS our responsibility.

Delving a little deeper into the possible causes of neglect, I found the following as the most relevant:

1- I do not feel capable.

2- I have no confidence that I am doing it well.

3- It didn't work in some situations.

4- I do not believe that Reiki can help in certain situations.

5- I do not believe in Reiki.

6- I simply forgot about it.

Of these six fundamental causes, the first two are directly relevant to a matter of faith. Doubt is installed on the mind of the Reiki practitioner, blocking all ability to experiment with the tool. The 1st cause is the crisis of faith in oneself, which is one of the most complexes to address. The 2nd is a combination of self-doubt and doubt in the process you are doing, in this case Reiki. These two causes are very common when you study Reiki from an emotional and experiential perspective that exalts and strengthens your faith in what you're studying. When we are in an emotional crisis, our faith is non-existent; we are emotionally unstable and cannot address things from this angle.

The 3rd and 4th causes most commonly associated with a biased interpretation of the experience. This is the case in which I have been using Reiki to get something and the result was not favorable to me. This usually breaks the faith in Reiki and makes the Reiki practitioner to letting go aside. If, emotional understanding of Reiki can also lead to this result, the same way that religious crises occur when the God in question does not meet personal expectations of the believer.

The 5th is not a crisis of faith. It is an undeniable claim that Reiki practitioner and Reiki have nothing to do together. Honestly, I only have seen this case once. It is very rare that someone who has been in contact with Reiki in any of its forms has not even a doubt about the good in it.

The 6th cause has to do explicitly with attention, the level of awareness and personal responsibility. It happened with more than one of my students of Reiki, which discuss with me about some past or present situation that ails them. I limit myself many times to ask: did you do Reiki?

Well, I have to say that often the answer is NO. I also recognize that in most of these cases, the person takes responsibility, starts sending Reiki and then harvest the results from an appropriate level of consciousness.

*I wanted to cultivate myself spiritually, to know everything in order to find what I like and specialize. I asked my teacher where to start and she told me learn Reiki. In theory I liked the potential of Reiki, but in practice, although I feel that it works, I don't think it is my calling. The truth is that astrology and numerology most attracts my attention. Maybe I'm not a physical but psychological healer. That is the reason why I did not continue practicing, so I lost a little confidence in myself...*

You expose very clearly your relationship with Reiki.

I think like you. For each person there are tools more akin to others. Numerology and astrology tend to be widely accepted, as are very aware of the rational aspect that is so prevalent in these yang civilizations of left brain. So you use the left brain as a cane that helps you walk the path to your right brain. That is, going hand in hand with the rational to the intuitive. Once you grab confidence, probably you drop the cane and take flight with your intuition.

In Reiki this process is not even necessary, because it is not necessary for you neither to rationalize nor to perceive what the patient has. There is not diagnosis, but direct and simple balance, invoking universal love.

Reiki action is not only physical. In fact the results are much more noticeable in the mental and emotional spheres. So if you like to treat these areas, I recommend that occasionally you try Reiki. If you want you may start with someone with insomnia or something like that, so you can see the effect achieved.

Given the need we have to use the left hemisphere, in my classes I appeal to the energetic understanding of how Reiki works, so our rational side does not feel overshadowed by this technique and accepts it as useful and understandable.

*I am convinced that we are not the ones with healing powers. In my case, when I channel energy I do not feel like having any special powers, but having the grace to cross paths with this technique and I feel I am one arm directed by the transcendent.*

Yes, as you say is perfect. I feel the same as you.

What happens is that when I speak of these things the different egos intersect. For me there is a ego-self which is what has no power itself. It is what gives us the ability to believe we are separate from everything and everyone. Of course, with that cover letter that ego-self cannot get very far in the process of healing.

There is also a higher-self which is our highest aspect, angelic or divine, of which we are not fully aware and from which we feel we are separated thanks to the ego-self. It's all part of the game we choose when incarnating. This higher-self, which is our true essence, has all the ability to harmonize and heal our bodies on the physical plane. Of course, for this to happen, we must learn to put aside some aspects of the ego-self that limits us to fully connect with the higher-self. The magic of Reiki is based in facilitating that process by initiating reconnection. The rest is homework.

As to heal others, is totally impossible, because we are in a plane where the only rule is always in effect is free will. What the healers do is to create an atmosphere of harmony and balance such that it allows the patient to start his own healing. This decision is more or less conscious and sometimes even relates to his life plan.

Here, some questions answered from the perspective of ego-self and the Higher-Self:

| Question | Ego-Self | Higher-Self |
|---|---|---|
| Can I balance others? | YES | YES |
| Can I heal others? | YES | NO |
| Can I balance myself? | YES | YES |
| Can I heal my bodies? | NO | YES |

These questions can be a bit sketchy, but I explain them just to clarify a bit the previous idea.

*I recently did my 1st Reiki workshop, I really liked the course, but in the process of the cleansing energy, I felt very fragile emotionally, passing from anger to tears with amazing ease. My emotional weakness has affected my behavior and relationships. Now I have many questions like the following: Does Reiki really heal? What does it cures of? Is it necessary to go through suffering to then move to higher energy levels or "born again"? Do these effects are a result of poor practice of Reiki? I do not know ... I doubt about the positive results of Reiki.*

I see you're experiencing some events that might relate to Reiki and I think appropriate to remark some things:

The energy cleansing process of 21 days which includes, among other things, performing daily self-Reiki should not be interrupted. The irregularities in this process can stop the purges taking place, leaving them halfway. In this case we recommend restarting the process from day 1.

On many occasions autosuggestion may play us a trick. It is true that some purification processes present symptoms and Reiki masters are responsible for alerting about that. But this does not mean that inevitably have to be symptoms.

The purification process is as intense as that to be balanced. There are people with few emotional contrasts that just feel effects at this level, but they can feel big symptoms at physical or mental level. People with a very ample emotional aspect, are likely to experience a big alternation in their emotions, as part of their own setting.

As for your questions, I can give you my own opinion, but only your insight can give you an answer that is appropriate for you.

*Does Reiki really heal?* No, it does not heal. Healing is done by the person by mechanisms that we can only guess. Reiki balances the energy bodies (physical, ethereal, emotional and mental). The person is responsible for maintaining this balance in its everyday life, with its attitudes and its levels of attention and awareness

*What does it cures of?* To cure, unlike healing, can be understood as alleviate symptoms. In this case, the balancing action of Reiki manages to harmonize the energies of the physical and etheric, improving the perception of symptoms. This can go further and become a true healing, if the patient is involved in the process at some level.

*Why feeling so bad and then feel good? Is it necessary to go through suffering to then move to higher energy levels or "born again"?* It is not mandatory to feel bad and then "reborn", but each person lives these processes on its own way. I did not feel bad with Reiki initiations, except occasional gastrointestinal symptoms in the first level. I know of cases with no symptoms ever and others who experience all kinds of things. Each process is personal and has no case to generalize the experience. What you feel, is not due to Reiki, but to your own energy configuration when making the initiation as well as the way you've done your energy cleansing.

*Do these effects are a result of poor practice of Reiki?* Like I said before, if you have not done your 21 days properly you may have open processes that have not been closed. In the end, it's your relationship with Reiki what determines the outcome.

I do not know ... I doubt about the positive results of Reiki. The "positive" results are as likely as the "negative" and both have their role in our life processes. Reiki only balances. The rest is our perception and judgment of the facts.

Anyway, no tool or system is "good for everyone". We are individuals, which mean that we are unique and therefore there is not one thing "good for everyone". Reiki may not be working for you. But it seems to me that it is working on you quite well and its effects are scaring you. Apparently you are removing some certainties and defenses to which you have become used to face the world. That can happen and scares. Of course I'm just speculating.

I recommend you do not stop working with self-Reiki and take into account the principles of Reiki in your life.

I feel a little bit ashamed, but I think this is the opportunity to comment and I understand. I did the first level of Reiki, I practiced alone with me, because I feel shame to tell other people, I tried at home and they accepted but as to please me and that discouraged me so no longer practiced it.

*I feel like a need to do it, sometimes I feel a tingling in my hands and I do it to myself or plants and the need goes away. Does this mean that after one is attuned, the energy starts to flow and you need to practice?*

Good that you got the courage to share your experience. Look, once you start you are a Reiki channel and Reiki channels get warm hands or get tingling with no apparent reason. Sometimes, just talking about Reiki makes you feel the heat in your hands.

You are not required to practice Reiki nor will you receive no punishment if you don't do it. But have you given any thought to the huge potential you have being attuned into Reiki? Do you remember what moved you first to do Reiki and the magic of initiation? What a waste of that wonderful energy to disconnect from it, right?

For me, what you do is very good. Whenever you feel that tingling let yourself go with your intuition and impose hands on your body, the other's, a plant, an animal, etc.

If people sometimes do not ask for Reiki or you think they ask for it just to please you, it is because you feel some fear and insecurity with the technique and results.

It has happened with several students that I have received with a level I and when they resume Reiki, the reaction of family and friends is of greater acceptance. This is because they themselves have been accepted as Reiki practitioners.

If at first they draw back with excuses and somehow ashamed for doing self-Reiki, after all relatives are watching their space and time for him to follow his sessions in peace and protect them from any distraction or interference.

It is a phenomenon that has much to do with what one projects. So practice a lot with yourself, feel the connection, rejoice your heart and remember that you are God. Reiki orders will come alone. You will see!

*I started with Reiki a month ago, being emotionally unstable, with a slight depression. I tend to doubt myself, whether I'm doing it correctly or not. Some days I feel very connected others I wake up slightly melancholic and somewhat hard for me to connect with the beauty of Reiki. Despite my self-esteem issues I feel with all my heart that I'll be fine, because I know I am healing, slightly, but I do!*

Yes, it is as you say. In times of depression and low self-esteem, that's when one needs Reiki, but then confidence falters and we decide to lay hands.

It's beautiful what you're doing with yourself. First, you have become aware of things you do not like, what do you want to change and then, you have committed to change. In addition, you agree that this change occurs in time, at its pace, so it is done in depth, not superficially. I think large part of the battle is won with that attitude. Just be perseverant and everything will be fine. Remember that Reiki is not a matter of faith. It is energy, is always energy and the nature of the energy is to flow.

## Can Reiki regenerate evicted nerve tissue?

*I wonder if Reiki can stimulate or activate the regeneration of nerve tissue seriously damaged, to be more precise, "separated".*

I think Reiki can really support the creation of miracles, given that the miracle is always performed by the very "patient" (it is ironic that is called patient if it's the one doing all the work, right?)

In my particular experience, I attuned a person in Reiki who suffered with multiple sclerosis. You know it's a disease where the nerves lose their covering and short-circuits are produced between nerve signals. This brings great problems of coordination at all levels, motor, mental, etc. With time comes to affect the functioning of the autonomic nervous system to such an extent that affects the vital functions and compromises the life of the person.

This person, after initiation, began to regain her mental coordination, to recover the memory that she was losing, to better coordinate the movements, and her life quality improved greatly. The question of whether nerve sheath was recovered with Reiki, I cannot answer. But the result speaks for itself.

I think that the injured person can get benefits from Reiki for recovery, but the key ingredients are to be constant and not doubt your ability to heal.

Reiki promotes a state of equilibrium such in our bodies, which allows expression of the power of self-healing. If the person chooses to take sessions with someone it would help her a lot; and if she also feels motivated to learn how to apply it, so much the better.

## Reiki Inteligent Energy

*I've heard that Reiki energy is intelligent. Does this make sense? Is not intelligence a human attribute?*

Regarding intelligent energy ... I think intelligence perhaps is not the right word, is it? Intelligence is just an expression of our limitations, although not enough. Wise certainly sounds better, because wisdom does not depend on knowledge, perceptions or physical plane. And the best of all, you do not even need to explain things.

Calling Reiki energy intelligent has to do, among other things, with:

- The ability that it has to locate itself where it "should"
- The absence of polarization of this energy
- The ability to act in accordance with our intention
- The ability to act independently of our intention
- The ability to remove time and space barriers
- Immateriality

Sure the list could be much longer, but these points can be a good starting point to begin with that which makes us perceive the Reiki energy as "smart".

*I have heard that "With our mind -disbelief, rationality- and our emotions -fear, mistrust- we can block or sabotage any energy work". Wouldn't this be a higher will causing the blocking?*

It's probably as you say, but in the midst of all this game, the only rule we usually leave out is the free will. The sleeping human is a victim of all the circumstances, while the master is an awake human handling all circumstances. It is a matter of level of consciousness that does not rest outside, nor above, but within us.

## Experience of Distant Attunement

I have practiced Remote Reiki treatments by sending energy at different latitudes and clients with varying degrees of understanding about energy healing. That's why I can say that in Reiki, distance is not an obstacle for the healing process to work. I have even noticed that for some clients the perception and impact of Reiki is greater at distance than that in presence.

Almost a year ago a door to my practice of Reiki opened, something I had not considered seriously before: the distant Reiki attunements. It all started with a friend who lives in Europe. His father was sick and asked me to attune her. His father was also my friend, so almost without thinking, I chose to listen to my heart and I ended up doing the attunement.

The relevance of this fact is that at that time the seed was sowed of something that nowadays has become a wonderful experience for me: Reiki attunements online.

Spurred by another friend who was attuned online, I've been training Reiki practitioners at distance, working on videoconferencing to provide visual contact during the process. The results obtained by the Reiki practitioners, both in their personal processes and treatment to others, have been significant and do not differ from the results obtained by my students in presence.

I would like to share this with you, in order to provide further evidence that Reiki, as for love, distance is not a limitation.

# MY STUDENTS SPEAK

## Francesca

Trying to tell you what we can become through Reiki is not so simple, simply because we are facing an energy experience that constantly transforms and renews us, making us live the reality in a different way and can hardly be explained only through words.

There are just 2 months I am attuned with this so beautiful energy and every day I am grateful for letting myself to enjoy this gift. Until now, the most important experiences I have lived are on a personal level. By this I mean that while applying Reiki I have had very good results with people, animals and plants, the experience within me has been even more intense, because this is definitely an energy that acts first on our consciousness and then, with the power of our intention is manifested above all else. I tell you some episodes.

First Level. The first few weeks were not easy. The attunement experience was like getting the most important emotional slap of my life. In those ten minutes it lasted, I felt I was cleaning inside from everything disturbing me over the last years, including feelings which until then I had not been able to recognize.

The 21 days of cleansing, I was synchronizing with what I would call "the other reality". It's like if you start experiencing things and people from another perspective. You feel like your everyday continues its normal rhythm, but your inner world is no longer the same, definitely moves at a different rhythm You are not separated from your reality, but inwardly you start living with detachment, with objectivity, with more awareness. It's as if you'll adjust the hands of your internal clock and move them forward just a couple of seconds, allowing you to react to all stimuli in a completely different way, I would say, proactive.

This experience has led me to feel an emotional peace that each day takes better form. It's not easy to look like this (from the inside out) because we are used precisely to the opposite. And one can then be tempted to start making excuses for not going forward with Reiki. We also have to have great courage to accept within us something so beautiful and simple and not sabotage well-being moments replacing them with problems; mechanisms we use to draw the attention of others, which often give "good" results but at the expense of our health.

If we are going to help others, we must first take responsibility for ourselves and that's the wonderful thing about Reiki because once you tune into your true self, the mask falls off.

Second Level Notes. I arrived very well to the course. However, attunement again started acting out but this time physically. I ended the training with 38.5°C (101.3 ° F) fever and a mental state that I would not been able to solve the simplest sum. The fever took away only the day the group performed distant healing that we had established as a method of daily practice on each of us. I was with fever, sinusitis and general malaise for about 1 week. I had the first migraine of my life and from there everything started to change for the better. I must say that even in the worst of moments my sessions of self-Reiki and distance healing were interrupted.

With this level I felt like I was constantly absent.

During the 21 day cleanse, in some self-Reiki practices, I had several very beautiful episodes that consisted of experiencing microseconds of profound and intense happiness. Not even the best words can describe them. There simply be lived.

And Aristides was right when he told us in his lectures that this energy is available to all. He transmits it so naturally and spontaneously that I doubted it was possible to tune without much effort and without having to become an "Enlightened One" or something.

Thanks to Aristides and everyone with whom I shared this experience that is just beginning and from which I'm starting to feel the benefits in every aspect of my life.

## Cecilia Camargo

For me Reiki has been a window to peace. At first I could not be consistent with it, but when I did I felt different. It solved my problems in a different way and from the heart; every way I feel better , I have more patience and I know that is an effective tool in every moment of my life. I have helped friends and family and I feel closer to God. I feel I am a simple tool with which it works to help others.

## Mimi Urrunaga

Master Dunas arrives into my life and is through Reiki that a transformation starts, not only professionally because I already had been working for years in therapy, but first and foremost, on a personal level.

In our work together and so devoted from his part (that I will never be thankful enough), a big change begins to operate on me, what he calls the levels of consciousness: being able to be awake, being able to be here and now and being capable to achieve consistency between feeling, thinking and acting. Daring to break even the most entrenched of the schemes and concepts that I could feel tied up, until a profound change in me took effect and therefore, this change begins to change my life and that of my loved ones. I soon realized that not only I and my world were being transformed, but my conception of life itself, had changed, is changing...

Naturally all this leads to a radical and wonderful change in my therapeutic work techniques and so the people who have been under my treatments have seen the benefits, very quickly and yet very subtle, because Reiki works in a way so wise there is no way in which there is no answer. I have seen, just as I first saw it in myself, how people treated, make a great bright and positive change in their consciousness levels in the physical, the emotional, spiritual. And I have seen with emotion changes in their lives and with a smile on their faces, almost without any effort.

Dunas and Reiki teachings are a permanent change; they are one being the most alert possible to see the miracle and magic of life itself.

I experienced the miracle in my three levels of Reiki, after beautiful, almost magical life experiences, in each of the attunements I received. Learning that there is no distance, no limits for light and energy, there is no obstacle to the commitment and dedication of a good teacher that the gods put in my destiny.

I've been able to work with Dunas in several remote attunements, in very different persons and with different types of life, faith and expectations before Reiki and seen in all great changes. It will be the moment for the master and them to make comments to this respect.

I will say that when witnessing attunements I have lived so intense and beautiful experiences that few would be the words I can find to describe that. Next to Dunas I've seen transformation of lives; opening of new universes ... I still see subtle changes.

We have learned with Dunas and traveling companions how to transform and love each other with a real and unconditional love to ourselves, as a human group, not being the distance and time a limitation. I have seen and lived in myself great friendships, great brotherhoods and great laughter, since we have also learned to laugh and laugh out loud. I have seen the magic, alchemy and transmutation.

We have seen and accompanied the birth and death of human beings, being with them in the process. We have seen several who thought they were finished for the art of living coming back to life.. We have seen the rebirth of dreams, illusions and hopes. We have been able to be reborn.

Namaste Master Dunas! Namaste to life and to masters guiding me. Here begins a new path.

## Joana Braca

Reiki is a portal to many dimensions, is like unconditional love (always there, by and for all and free), it is a privilege, a blessing, an awakening of consciousness, a new dawn. With Reiki I: became aware of my body: now I do not smoke, I don't eat red meat or poultry; I use alcoholic beverages, only for what I choose because now I do it consciously. Reiki II: was a hurricane rose, removed everything from my guts (strong emotional level), but it filled all with love and gave me hope and one more reason to live. Reiki III: "simple" but more powerful than a tsunami, just thinking and creates a state of healing. The most moving anecdote was curettage (mini surgery) applied to a young girl with a drop of several steps and bruised hip. It had to be quick because there was no other way, curettage was performed no more than 5 minutes: hematoma and as we say in colloquial "the bump", disappeared instantly, was miraculous. Reiki is my transporting vehicle and my great love.

## Haydeé Belisario

Last year I had the good fortune to be initiated into Reiki. If you ask me what has become Reiki for me? I would just tell you that being in harmony with this Divine Energy allowed me to understand how easy it is to live and it is us who complicate our existence with all the misconceptions we have stored.

Reiki has helped me in such an imperceptible yet so palpable way that almost without realizing it has wrought changes in my life than previously believed unattainable. Events that have happened to me at another time would have said "are incredible". Now I know that in everything that happens there are things to learn and pass precisely because it is the only way to grow spiritually and overcome these apparent limitations.

Raising our level of consciousness allows us to live each day with pleasure "knowing that everything has a solution", dedicating ourselves to what we do with gratitude and love.

Finally I give thanks to the Universe, to my teacher of Reiki Aristides Molina and all those who guided me towards the study of Reiki because they let me get in tune with something that just is WONDERFUL. With Love.

## Marinela Ramírez

My Reiki experience: I met Aristides Molina when collaborating with his newspaper Canal de Luz (Channel of Light). I read his articles on Reiki and other matters; we talked about many subjects while watching his attitude to people, situations and learning. I realized that Reiki was "something" fundamental that I had been missing; that what I had read and discussed with Reiki practitioners was not enough to capture its essence and that it was much more than a mere technique: an attitude towards life, a different way of feeling the energy of the universe and flow with it. I signed up for the next Attunement with the certainty that I would learn something important, yet did not know what but my rational side was telling me that surely the experience would finish there. However, my contact with Reiki moved many schemes in me and opened me up to a new dimension of energy which had not acceded to with Universal Energy, Flower Therapy, Dowsing or Meditation I had cultured for more than 20 years. As a result, I went ahead and, after 21 days of self-Reiki, got ready to receive the Attunement of the Second Level, after which followed another

21 days of practice even more intense and my motivation for continuing with the Third Level. Each attunement exceeds my expectations by far and enriches me personally, emotionally and spiritually.

Pursuing this loving contact with me, with the other, with the universe, I've experienced inner opening, a guide that marks the way to move forward. I have a greater state of alert, I have made significant personal fulfillment as the strengthening of my relationship, through marriage. I have increased my ability to give and receive love; I am open to prosperity and have started editing books that I had been writing for seven years. My first book (on Tarot and self-knowledge) hits the market while this one.

To date I am already registered to continue with Reiki Mastery, with the certainty that this will awaken something still asleep within me providing me with scenarios for growth and inner alchemy I'll be conscious and willing to accept, like never before. Namaste.

## Beatriz Lozano

My experience with Reiki I and II has been and continues to be a positive and amazing experience from any angle, from where we focus. Everything continues happening every day ... Definitely, something happened to me since I started with Dunas and that something that happens every day, I feel it reflected in what I do, whether small or great, important or trivial. I can feel it in my relationships with others and with myself.

I understand myself more, I love myself more, even people on the street smiles at me for no apparent reason! and I still am in the process, practicing, because I know I'm just getting started, discovering a new universe, but actually walking, lighter, more aware, happier ... simply living Reiki.

## Yanira Molina

When master Dunas asked me to write a testimonial about what Reiki "did" for me, I said without hesitation, of course, is a breeze, but when I sat down to write I went blank. How to write about subtle but profound changes that allowed the "Reiki energy" made in my life? As the Tao that can be expressed in words is not the true Tao, Reiki and its influence that can be expressed in words is not the real Reiki, here is an approximation.

To begin with the arrival of this energy into my life was very causal. From the moment I heard about it I thought it was one of the many follies of my father, who was in a process of changing his life and as I was "comfortable" with mine, I had nothing to do with it. Within months, talking to my dad about what were we going to drink with our dinner, I felt certain that I wanted "this thing of Reiki" and from that moment I changed profoundly.

Before Reiki I was a person with many emotional obstacles, many fears that were hidden under a thick mask that made them completely unknown to me. After Reiki they all went away ... it is a lie. Reiki helped me (and still does) to thin the mask slowly allowing me to see through it, discovering the many facets of my being that good or bad, are part of me, and making me more aware of whom I am. The road for me just begun and I am filled with GRATITUDE having this tool so beautiful.

## Siomara Gálvez

"Reiki is a gift of love given to us by the universe," said my teacher Aristides starting the talk of the attunement. I totally agree with him and I express my infinite gratitude with all my heart. .

It happens that I started as a patient, suffering from insomnia for several years. I told Aristides by chance and he suggested that I were about to get "something" for several days at night. With total disregard for what it was I laid quietly on agreed time. At that moment I had a warm feeling that once hugged me and pulled me, followed by sounds of small bells in a short peal. Then I fell asleep. From this wonderful event it's been three years that I sleep without difficulty.

This experience leaned my compass in the quest to find that "something" that had happened to me, so I asked consciously to be attuned into the knowledge and practice of that resource. I am currently in level II and during this period I have taken Reiki as a valuable experience in my day to day. Its constant practice gives me confidence and peace in solving my challenges, resulting in a change in perception and manifestation of my life. It's like using a marker and says before and after Reiki.

The experience through Reiki make me much more aware about the potential we have to manifest what we want, using Reiki as a tool to focus and allow our choice.

## Graciela Zerpa Urbina

My experience with Reiki. When I thought about Reiki, I asked myself: What do I want this for?, I do not see myself on a stretcher giving the treatment, it is a rare thing; it is simply hands-on, is the same as for a man that I know, and I do not need it, I have my work. What I like is Astrology and I don't identify myself with Japanese ideology. At that time all that appeal to me was attending courses, one after the other. I did not know what I wanted. Each time had more information but I was very confused, empty and sad. But one day I noticed a change in my sister-in-law that, from being someone extremely methodical with her life and live every week in a clinic or hospital for asthma treatment, I found her totally relaxed, happy and looked like ten years younger, besides attracting me to be with her and talk to her all the time.

At that same time I was getting to know Aristides and I attended a talk, but I had no idea what it was, I simply went to hear the information. In one hour he made an impression on me and automatically in December 2004 followed the first level of Reiki. It was magic from the start. I felt as if flows of energy run through my body from head to toe. Then I observed that by dropping my arms, they did not touch my body, it was like that bounced and bounced. On the other hand, when resting my hands sleeping I felt as if they were floating on the mattress and felt wow! That feeling is so divine. At that moment I thought that Reiki was only sensory.

Day after day I continued practicing self-healing, until I started to feel better and be less dependent on medicines, painkillers and books to find answers everywhere. I realized that I was more relaxed, I crashed the car and got out and instead of wanting to kill the man that struck me (as was usual in me) that event do not even bother me. I was happier with myself, my family and my friends. Improved my relationship and I began to accept the world as it is and feel that everything is in perfect harmony.

I noted on the street that everyone was smiling and gave me a good morning, they assisted me in good shape and everything in my life flowed by magic. Then I realized that Reiki was not a hobby, a job or something that was going to practice from time to time, but now Reiki was me, it is all around me, is a way of life with its own ecosystem. Now every time I meet someone looking for that magic answer of life, and feeling uneasy about this "I don't know what", that makes us feel empty and unhappy although we have everything we wanted in this life; I recommend that before any therapy, personal growth, holistic, esoteric experiential workshop or course, etc., they start being attuned in Reiki and feel that the doors of all they want to develop in their lives is going to open in a magical and perfect way. My personal opinion is that Reiki was the first step to feel alive.

Thank you. Namaste.

## Miriam Coronado

While I and II initiations were received with great love and receptivity, the III was the one that marked something different, so I would share this beautiful work of my teacher Aristides Molina:

1- During the attunement three Buddha Masters manifested. I understand they are my ruling masters for working with Reiki. Finalized this stage received the following:

"That I have travelled has been more than walking the tracks left in other times and places. Learning and unlearning to find the ends of the cycle is getting completed, this is the objective of the journey lived in each attunement. Overcoming the will of the ego by the divine will is to find the humility and simplicity of heart that dwells in each disciple of the path of initiation, which is the Great Treasure that is installed on each initiate".

2- When I got home after finishing the years after this third initiation, I began to feel I was in two dimensions at the same time. I quieted the interpretation that this was part of the set of frequencies that surely had happened during this attunement. The experience, although it is the second time this happens to me (the first was in another attunement), demand from us temperance and conviction of what is happening, since it is not easy to see and feel that at the same time the occurrence of events with apparent different realities. It's like reading this book while you are playing with a ball at the beach. After three hours it lasted, my reflection was that the energy spread out by the use of Antahkarana may have helped in this parallel experience of dimensions.

With love and blessings,

## Dra. Rossbi Infante

I've really had many testimonials thank God and my day to day is to be a vehicle for direct and distance healing. But I find this case very interesting where a lady had a right breast cancer formed by a dense ball. We practice several Reiki treatments on her and after some days she got another mammogram and there was no need to operate as the lump in his breast had diminished. That experience was wonderful and as such there are others but this was the one that has made a greater impression in me visually. Every action must take place with a lot of faith and especially when healing.

## Grecia Palma

What a joy to share with you what Reiki has done in my life. Reiki is Love and it has transformed my life, helping me to fortify me, to grow, to love-live. And what is to live?

To live is imagining and dreaming. To live is feeling and believing. It is also thinking, saying and listening. To live is to believe in oneself and in others. It is to give and to share. To live is crying and laughing. To live is the most valued gift God has given us. To live makes me the Owner of the Sun and the air, of the sky and winds, of the mountains and the stars. Reiki made me owner of myself and my decisions. In short, what I am and I intend to be.

## Yanira Herrera

On a personal level I have used Reiki to balance my emotions. On the first level there was strong evidence at family level, especially because I was regaining control of my life. The second level also moved great deal of the emotional part. I think that every work on the planet is rooted on emotions and transcend is given there. A person came into my life with the "vice" of controlling relationships. In other circumstances, I might have got carried away, but I realized that I was driven over there and realized that I do not want a controlling relationship, but to share from the heart and uninhibited.

With the symbols a curious thing happened. I'm on the street waiting for a bus and I see a very sick puppy. He was walking on three legs, crawling. I concentrate myself for a moment and made the symbol of strength. A few seconds later the dog approaches me walking perfectly on all fours with excellent face. It was a great impression!

My daughter's case is interesting. She fell and the doctors said she had to go through a surgery of the right knee. I searched the Antahkarana mandalas and started working with them. I made a total of 5 treatments. I also used acupuncture four times and spent four days with the splint. When an MRI was taken, the result was that surgery was not needed and she was walking perfectly. The MRI showed as if the lesion had healed.

# ABOUT THE AUTHOR

Arístides Molina (Dunas) is an Engineer, Reiki Master, Therapist and Life Coach, specialized in personal activation processes and emotional management.

In his path of personal development, Reiki has always been one of its fundamental pillars.

He has trained hundreds of therapists in Reiki, Tapping, Life Mastery and other disciplines, in different countries of America and Europe.

More about the autor:
http://estoesreiki.com
http://aristidesmolina.com

If you feel this book has given you a better understanding of Reiki and its possibilities; I'd appreciate your comments at Amazon for others, like you, also benefit from the ideas in this book.

Sharing is creating and growing.

Thank you in advance for supporting the Reiki community.